A GRASSROOTS HISTORY

— OF THE —

HIV/AIDS EPIDEMIC

IN NORTH AMERICA

OTHER BOOKS OF INTEREST FROM MARQUETTE BOOKS

John Markert, *The Social Impact of Sexual Harassment: A Resource Manual for Organizations and Scholars* (2010). ISBN 978-0-9826597-4-8 (paperback)

John C. Merrill, *Farewell to Freedom: Impact of Communitarianism on Individual Rights in the 21st Century* (2011).
ISBN: 978-0-9826597-5-5 (paperback)

John W. Cones, *Introduction to the Motion Picture Industry: A Guide for Students, Filmmakers and Scholars* (2009).
ISBN: 978-0-922993-90-1 (paperback)

John Schulz, *Please Don't Do That! The Pocket Guide to Good Writing* (2008).
ISBN: 978-0-922993-87-1 (booklet)

Global Communication Association and the Global Fusion Consortium, *Global Media Journal: Volumes 1-3 and 3-5* (2008). ISBNs: 978-0-922993-69-7 and 978-0-922993-70-3 (paper)

Héctor Luis Díaz, Johnny Ramírez-Johnson, Randall Basham and Vijayan K. Pillai, *Strengthening Democracy Through Community Capacity Building* (2008). ISBN: 978-0-922993-95-6 (paper)

John W. Cones, *Dictionary of Film Finance and Distribution: A Guide for Independent Filmmakers* (2008). ISBN: 978-0-922993-93-2 (cloth); 978-0-922993-94-9 (paper)

Hazel Dicken-Garcia and Giovanna Dell'Orto, *Hated Ideas and the American Civil War Press* (2008). ISBN: 978-0-922993-88-8 (paper); 978-0-922993-89-5 (cloth)

Mitchell Land and Bill W. Hornaday, *Contemporary Media Ethics: A Practical Guide for Students, Scholars and Professionals* (2006). ISBN: 0-922993-41-6 (cloth); 0-922993-42-4 (paperback)

Stephen D. Cooper, *Watching the Watchdog: Bloggers as the Fifth Estate* (2006).
ISBN: 0-922993-46-7 (cloth); 0-922993-47-5 (paperback)

David Demers, *Dictionary of Mass Communication: A Guide for Students, Scholars and Professionals* (2005). ISBN: 0-922993-35-1 (cloth); 0-922993-25-4 (paperback)

A GRASSROOTS HISTORY

— OF THE —

HIV/AIDS EPIDEMIC

IN NORTH AMERICA

JAMES GILLETT

MARQUETTE BOOKS LLC
SPOKANE, WASHINGTON

Printed in the United States of America

Library of Congress Cataloging Number
2010938482

ISBN for this edition:
978-0-9826597-7-9

Background cover photo
Copyright 2006 Martin Haase
Used with permission
fotolio.com

Marquette Books LLC
3107 East 62nd Avenue
Spokane, Washington 99223
509-443-7057 (voice) / 509-448-2191 (fax)
books@marquettebooks.com / www.MarquetteBooks.com

For Meghan, Rebecca, Hannah and Jasper

CONTENTS

INTRODUCTION

In 1981, the Centre for Disease Control and Prevention (CDC) reported cases of a rare form of pneumonia and cancer usually only associated with diminished immune function among gay men living in large urban areas in the United States (Gilman, 1988). In *Outreach*, the publication of the San Francisco AIDS Foundation, it is noted that the cases were mentioned in the *New York Times* and the *San Francisco Chronicle* highlighting the seriousness of the disease and its prevalence among gay men (AIDS at 25, 2006). A year after the CDC announcement, the diagnostic category AIDS, or acquired immune deficiency syndrome, was given to categorize the illness that was spreading at an alarming rate, primarily among gay men. By the end of 1982, more than 600 people had died AIDS-related deaths in the United States (American Association for World Health, 2001). The institutional response to AIDS in the early 1980s was essentially nonexistent given the gravity of the epidemic, despite an awareness of AIDS among those in the CDC and the mass media. Organizing among gay men and lesbians in response to the epidemic offered the only support and education services available and was a crucial form of early advocacy about HIV/AIDS (Altman, 1986). In the context of this community-based response, many of the gay men diagnosed with AIDS refused to adopt the conventional patient role of compliance and subservience to institutional authority. Instead, building on the political tenets of the gay and lesbian movement and the women's health movement, they mobilized and demanded to be involved in the policies, services, and organizations that were emerging to deal with the epidemic.

This initial organizing during the early 1980s in Canada and the United States led to a much broader political movement among people with HIV/AIDS. Over the last twenty-five years, those infected with HIV/AIDS — combined with the support and involvement of those directly affected by the disease — have organized to provide mutual support, education and advocacy. People with HIV/AIDS — also often referred to as People Living with HIV/AIDS and using the acronym PWA or PHA — have come together collectively around the common experience of living with a disease in order to become actively involved in the decisions that affect their lives. A central vehicle for this activism has been and continues to be the formation of local, regional, national and international organizations. The National Association of People with AIDS (NAPWA), for instance, began as an initiative of a small group of activists in 1983 during the formative years of the People with AIDS (PWA) self-empowerment movement. NAPWA continues to do advocacy work, raise awareness, offer community development programs, and facilitate social networking for individuals with HIV/AIDS and PWA organizations. The continuation of NAPWA, and the formation of global and international PWA networks (like the Global Network of People Living with HIV/AIDS or GNP+), is a testament to the ongoing efforts to mobilize among people with HIV/AIDS.

In his book *Power and Community*, Altman (1994) argues that the community-based response to HIV/AIDS has been effective and subversive because "it has challenged the expert control of knowledge and the state's control of policy" (p.1). In many respects, organizing by and for people with HIV/AIDS has been at the forefront of this challenge. Using strategies of self-empowerment, the PWA movement has encouraged and assisted the involvement of those infected in all decisions that affect their lives. Being involved has meant reworking and changing societal norms and assumptions about what it means to live with an infectious, life-threatening disease. The purpose of this book is to chart the historical trajectory of organizing and activism by people living with HIV/AIDS during four key moments in the epidemic in North America between 1983 and 2008.

Understanding Organizing and Activism by People with HIV/AIDS

Over the last twenty-five years, the voices and actions of people with HIV/AIDS have been an integral component of the community-based response to the epidemic. Yet, the involvement of HIV positive individuals in PWA organizing and activism has received limited direct scholarly attention (Roy & Cain, 2001). Early critical accounts of the epidemic, like Altman's (1986) *AIDS in the Mind of America* or Cindy Patton's (1985) *Sex and Germs*, paid limited attention to the early PWA self-empowerment movement as a component of the community mobilization that emerged in the face of widespread stigma, moral panic and institutional neglect. People with HIV/AIDS acting collectively were portrayed primarily as self-help initiatives providing practical assistance and support. Patton (1990) describes early PWA organizing as:

> a hybrid between a gay liberation/identity model and the lobby/self-help model of such health-related groups as the Multiple Sclerosis Society ... , which similarly create micro-cultures of diverse people sharing a common medically-related experience. (p. 10)

In this scholarship, the political significance of mobilization among people with HIV/AIDS was secondary to challenging the emergent discourses of homophobia and fear that characterized early public perceptions of the disease and influenced the development of policy and programs, which, as a result, ran counter to preventing the spread of HIV/AIDS among communities most at risk (Watney, 1987).

Writing about the place of people with HIV/AIDS in political organizing and activism began to emerge in the late 1980s with the rise in prominence of direct action groups like ACT UP and AIDS ACTION NOW! Out of this movement came a number of influential texts that were collaborative projects between artists, critics and activists. A key work was Douglas Crimp's 1988 edited collection for a special issue of the journal *October*, published afterward as the book, *AIDS: Cultural Analysis/Cultural Activism* (1988). This anthology broke with academic convention and created a pastiche of articles and images by activists, people with HIV/AIDS, artists, critics and academics. Of note is a series of articles by Max Navarre on the actions of people with HIV/AIDS to organize politically and challenge misconceptions about the disease. In the articles "Fighting the Victim Label" (1988) and "PWA Coalition Portfolio" (1988), Navarre describes the key tenets of PWA self-empowerment and organizing in the early 1980s. A number of edited anthologies on HIV/AIDS and cultural politics from this period similarly highlighted PWA organizations and the actions of people living with HIV/AIDS in articulating a critique of institutional AIDS representations, policies, and programs (Carter & Watney, 1989; Miller, 1992).

This writing sought to document and give prominence to emergent forms of cultural activism arising from the epidemic in the late 1980s (Crimp, 1990; 2004). The significance of art and cultural practices in contesting and reconstructing meanings associated with HIV/AIDS was a key theme throughout this literature. Attention to the identity and cultural politics in AIDS activism by artists, academics and cultural critics in the 1980s informed a line of inquiry in the social sciences in the 1990s on organizing among people with HIV/AIDS. One direction of this inquiry was the study of organizing and activism around access to and the availability of treatments for HIV/AIDS. Epstein's (1995; 1996) research explores the transformation of clinical medicine and medical research in response to pressure from AIDS activists. In his studies of knowledge construction and credibility in new social movements, Epstein (1995) highlights the historical significance of people with HIV/AIDS as lay experts in legitimating the efforts of treatment activism:

> But the AIDS movement is indeed the first social movement in the United States to accomplish the mass conversion of disease "victims" into activist-experts, and in that sense the AIDS movement stands alone, even as it begins to serve as a model for others. (p. 414)

The political mobilization of people with HIV/AIDS and their increased involvement in PWA organizations and AIDS organizations led to a renewed and vibrant treatment of activism in the 1990s. Strategies for chronic disease management and health promotion through a variety of means including allopathic and complementary medicine began the focal point of efforts around PWA self-empowerment and community development. Kahn (1993) documents the history of treatment activism during this period and attends to the actions of people with HIV/AIDS in forming health and treatment collectives in order to educate one another about health care options and gain access to difficult-to-obtain medications and therapies. PWA groups challenged the medical establishment in the use of experimental and alternative treatments through buyers clubs and community-based research. In an Australian context, Ariss & Dowsett (1997) similarly chart the development of treatment activism noting the lineage between the PWA self-empowerment movement in the 1980s and subsequent actions by activists and people with HIV/AIDS in 1990s. Treatment activism among those HIV infected sought to influence the state and health care systems regarding access to medical treatments and alternative therapies as a complement to conventional medical approaches.

Although still a minor line of inquiry, the advancement of "lay expertise" as a key concept legitimating the involvement of people with HIV/AIDS in organizing and activism led to studies examining the place of HIV positive individuals in the community-based response to the epidemic. In Canada, Roy (1995) conducted *Living and Serving,* a study exploring the contribution of people with HIV/AIDS to the AIDS movement and the barriers to their further involvement. This timely study coincided with a greater willingness among government officials and institutional authorities to acknowledge the need to include people with HIV/AIDS in decision-making processes. In 1994 at the Paris AIDS Summit, 42 countries agreed to the principle of the Greater Involvement of People Living with HIV/AIDS (GIPA), an initiative to increase the capacity of PWA organizations and include people with HIV/AIDS in decisions regarding policy and program development (UNAIDS, 2004). While recognized as valuable, it has only been in recent years that national and international agencies governments have embraced the GIPA principle, leading to greater support for PWA organizing and networks internationally (UNAIDS, 2004). Yet, research in this area continues to find significant and ongoing barriers to the involvement of people with HIV/AIDS in community-based organizations, policy development and research (Roy & Cain, 2001). A recent study by Travers et al. (2008)

found that while participation by people with HIV/AIDS is endorsed in principle, the capacity building and infrastructure necessary to facilitate this involvement in practice is lacking. Research on the application of the GIPA principle indicates a renewed interest in the contribution of people with HIV/AIDS in community organizing and public policy development (Maxwell et al., 2008). Attention to people with HIV/AIDS participating in organizing has extended to include research on initiatives internationally (Smith & Siplon, 2006; Seckinelgin, 2003).

Accompanying this interest in the involvement of people with HIV/AIDS in organizing and decision-making is research on the history of AIDS activism and the community-based response to the epidemic. Since the first identified cases, HIV/AIDS prompted social scientists and historians to consider the historical significance of the epidemic. Elizabeth Fee and Daniel Fox (1988; 1992) edited two key volumes charting the contemporary historiography of AIDS, the first (1988) on the early institutional depictions of the epidemic and the second (1992) on the shifting meaning of HIV/AIDS from terminal to chronic in the early 1990s. In this line of historical inquiry, sparked by works like Fee and Fox, few studies have explored the history of PWA organizing and activism (Herdt & Lindenbaum, 1992). More attention has been devoted to understanding the historical significance of direct action activist groups like ACT UP and AIDS ACTION NOW!

Of late, however, historians and scholars have begun to look back at the significance of activism over the course of the epidemic. A number of studies in this vein are local in orientation, concentrating the origins of activism in the epicenters of the epidemic in North America. Cochrane (2004) traces the beginnings of the epidemic in San Francisco from activist response to its initial surveillance and to the formation of knowledge about the disease that began during this initial period of the epidemic. Similarly, Maizel Chambré's (2006) recent book explores the beginning of the AIDS movement in New York, the other urban epicenter of the epidemic in the early 1980s. Brown (1997) adds to this historical work an understanding of early activism in Vancouver with an attention to the development of PWA organizations and direct action groups like ACT UP in this Canadian city. This scholarship shows the framing of AIDS activism in relation to specific locales, and together they provide a glimpse into the early history of the AIDS movement in North America. In addition to local studies are histories that take as their point of departure the life and writings of a single, prominent activist. Silversides' (2003) book on the life of AIDS activist Michael Lynch fits into this category. Silversides uses the diaries and writings by Lynch to reconstruct and analyze the origins and development of the early response to HIV/AIDS in Toronto and Canada.

Epidemic of Signification: Publishing By People with HIV/AIDS

This book builds upon prior efforts to understand organizing and activism by people with HIV/AIDS. Localized and activist histories of the HIV/AIDS epidemic signify an expanding interest in exploring the past three decades of the epidemic, especially from the perspective of those infected and affected. Like studies based on the reflections made by organizers and activists, my investigation draws on the writing by and for people with HIV/AIDS published in media developed in the context of the PWA organizing. The diaries of people like Michael Lynch, for instance, indicate a rich archive of material by people with HIV/AIDS on organizing and activism. As Duttmann (1996) has argued, the writings and reflections distilled from the experience of living with HIV/AIDS on one level make claims to an authentic representation of the epidemic but, more importantly, allow for the possibility of diverse narratives in which to render and account for this health crisis. One key feature of the PWA movement has been the print media forums that emerged from community-based organizations. PWA media projects foster cultures of survival through which people with HIV/AIDS sought political action, knowledge and information, social support and self-expression. This publishing offers a unique perspective on the epidemic not examined in the academic literature.

In looking at publishing by people with HIV/AIDS as a genre, I treat them as part of efforts among those involved in new social movements to construct a counter public sphere (Fraser, 1992). As Marshall (1991) has argued, contemporary social movements — feminism, environmentalism, gay liberation — have each created alternative public spheres through the use and development of communication media like print media, hotlines, videos, film, radio, and so on. Publishing in the context of a social movement serves as a counter public sphere on two levels. First, public forums allow people to share and articulate a critique of existing forms of domination. Secondly, they are a vehicle for articulating experiences and participate in the construction of a collective identity. As such, social movement media are counter-hegemonic. In developing public forums, people with HIV/AIDS provide mutual support and education otherwise not available. Furthermore, the opinions expressed in such forums become a way of influencing and challenging power structures that shape public policy decisions regarding HIV/AIDS.

PWA media projects have been integral to organizing by and for people with HIV/AIDS over the past fifteen years. The prevalence of such projects stems from the emphasis on staying informed as key strategy for survival within the PWA movement. The media projects used in this study generally fall into three categories: agency newsletters, treatment media, and magazines or zines. In the 1980s, when people with HIV/AIDS began to form their own organizations, they also started agency newsletters. The most notable, used extensively in this book, is *Newsline*, the publication of one of the first PWA organizations, the PWA Coalition of New York. *Body Positive* is a second key source of writing by people with HIV/AIDS. Until 2006, the organization Body Positive produced this agency newsletter that later would take on more of a magazine format. People with HIV/AIDS in New York in 1987 started the organization Body Positive to assist those who first acknowledged the impact of HIV/AIDS in their lives. The equivalent Canadian publication, *Living Positive*, began as the newsletter for the British Columbia Persons with AIDS Society, formerly the Vancouver PWA Coalition, formed in 1986. *Newsline, Living Positive*, and *Body Positive,* along with the numerous similar newsletters/magazines that have emerged over the years, help to document the history of PWA organizing and activism and the epidemic from the perspective of people with HIV/AIDS.

A second type of media project used in this book is AIDS treatment media. Founded and run by John S. James in 1986, the most notable treatment publication, *AIDS Treatment News*, has been providing information on a consistent basis relying primarily on subscriptions from readers. The content of *AIDS Treatment News* not only examines the medical side of health care but the social, political and public policy sides as well. As such, this publication is a valuable archival source of information about transformations that have occurred in PWA activism and the HIV health crisis. Unlike *AIDS Treatment News*, most treatment media are a service of community-based organizations. A second treatment media central to this book is *TAGline*, a publication of the Treatment Action Group (TAG). Formed in 1992, TAG works to "ensure that all people living with HIV receive the necessary treatment, care, and information they need to save their lives" (Treatment Action Group, n.d.). Over the last fifteen years, several prominent HIV positive treatment activists have written about health care, their lives and the epidemic in *TAGline*. Throughout the 1990s, many PWA and AIDS organizations created their own treatment publications featuring writing by people with HIV/AIDS. While many did not gain prominence nor last for any length of time, they still served as a source of information and a forum for dialogue and information about the medical and health care aspects of HIV/AIDS.

Along with treatment publications, another type of media project — zines and magazines about HIV/AIDS — emerged in the 1990s (Brouwer, 2005). This type of media project came about in part because people with HIV/AIDS with an interest in writing and in journalism started to produce their own publications. *Art and Understanding* is arguably the first "magazine about HIV/AIDS," started by David Waggoner in 1991 with the mandate to "save and archive the creative works of the HIV community." Not long after the start of *Art and Understanding*, a similar publication, *POZ Magazine*, followed with a glossy magazine format, though with a more political and current affairs point of reference. According to the magazine's HIV positive founder Sean Strub, *POZ* "sprang out of my desire to simplify, popularize and broadly disseminate the huge volume of life-sustaining information — and inspiration — I had already found critical to my own survival" (1997b). Counterposed to glossy magazines are zines — smaller, localized and independently produced publications created by small groups or collectives. While similar to magazines in that they attend to literary, political and cultural topics, zines follow an alternative rather than mainstream ethos. Of the numerous AIDS zines, *Diseased Pariah News* (*DPN*) and *Infected Faggot Perspectives* (*IFP*) have gained prominence as forums by and for people with HIV/AIDS that create a space for the expression of marginalized or silenced perspectives that challenge and contest conventional representations of the epidemic (Long, 2000; De Moor, 2005). Of the two, *Diseased Pariah News* had the greater longevity, beginning in 1991 and ending in 1999. A small group of HIV positive gay men started the zine to give voice to a more ironic, satirical, and pragmatic perspective on the disease; a voice that was missing or silenced in mainstream AIDS discourse. According to the founders, *DPN* is "a patently offensive publication of, by, and for people with HIV disease (and their friends and loved ones). We are a forum for infected people to share their thoughts, feelings, art, writing, and brownie recipes in an atmosphere free of teddy bears, magic rocks, and seronegative guilt."

Organization of the Book

The structure of this book mirrors significant trends in the trajectory of organizing and activism by people with HIV/AIDS. Over the last twenty-five years, the principle of self-determination and self-empowerment in the struggle to survive HIV/AIDS has been consistent through the PWA movement. The form of this organizing and activism by people with HIV/AIDS, however, has shifted in relation to transformations in the social, political, medical and epidemiological contours of the epidemic. In 2006, *Body Positive* published a timeline of the epidemic since the early 1980s that accurately reflects the trajectories of the movement identified and examined in this book.

Mobilization, 1983-89

After an initial period of uncertainty and confusion about the emergence of this new virus that was neither well understood nor seen to be a public policy priority, community organizers and activists began to mobilize collectively. PWA organizations along with the community-based AIDS movement more generally, emerged to address the needs of those infected and to challenge the panic and fear circulating in the mass media and by public officials. *Body Positive* described this period of protest as follows:

> Calls went out for mass quarantines, children with AIDS had their homes burned down, and AIDS phobic and homophobic attitudes skyrocketed. At the same time, people with AIDS grew ever more concerned and angered that no progress was being made on AIDS treatments. (Body Positive, 2006)

The first chapter examines the mobilization of people with HIV/AIDS between 1983 and 1989. Beginning with an account of the National AIDS Forum in Denver and the formulation of the basic principles of the PWA movement, I outline the historical context for organizing among those infected in the 1980s. Self-empowerment as the central strategy for encouraging people with HIV/AIDS to become involved in the decisions that affect their lives is the lens through which I examine significant moments during the early years of the movement. The sites for self-empowerment that emerged during this period of the epidemic include redefining the meaning of HIV, advocating for civil rights, acquiring the means for survival, and fostering social support and community development.

Normalization, 1989-1996

The second chapter of this book examines the period between 1989 and 1996. In the early 1990s PWA organizing and activism encountered an increasing normalization of the epidemic in North America. In the 1980s HIV/AIDS was highly stigmatized and social institutions did not effectively respond to the health crisis. While stigma remained a problem, in the 1990s there emerged a more concerted institutional response to the epidemic. The changing epidemiology of HIV/AIDS also contributed to the normalization of the epidemic. People with HIV/AIDS were living longer, healthier lives. The definition of HIV/AIDS as a chronic and manageable rather than terminal illness gained momentum during this period. Not only were people with HIV/AIDS living longer, the composition of the movement was also shifting. *Body Positive* characterized this period of normalization in the United States as follows:

> After the panic and protest of the late 1980s, AIDS starts to become "normalized." Fears over the possibility of casual transmission begin to fade and norms of safer sex become more established. People with HIV are protected from discrimination by the new Americans with Disabilities Act, and new funding commences for AIDS treatment. The announcement by basketball star Magic Johnson that he has HIV — while remaining healthy — redefines the disease in the minds of many. And the more progressive political approach adopted by the Clinton Administration calms protestors. But the death toll also continues to rise, and new treatments prove of limited value. (Body Positive, 2006)

After describing the institutional and activist response to the epidemic during this period, I trace a series of themes related to normalization that emerged from stories and portraits created by and for people living with HIV/AIDS. One predominate motif was portrayals of people with HIV/AIDS that emphasized the ordinary aspects of their lives. Ordinary in this sense is meant to "give HIV a human face" by highlighting the everyday lives of ordinary people who just happen to be HIV positive. A second theme emphasized the diversity, heterogeneity, and multiplicity of people with HIV/AIDS. Added to the images and writing of gay men were portraits of a much broader range of HIV-infected individuals and communities. I describe how the PWA movement continued to advance its central goals of ensuring that those infected were able to be involved in decisions that affected their lives — the idea of health from below — by responding to the increasing normalization of HIV/AIDS.

Medicalization, 1996-2000

The third chapter investigates a period of medicalization in the AIDS epidemic, beginning in 1996 at the International AIDS Conference in Vancouver. Results from clinical trials of a new class of medications called protease inhibitors changed the landscape of HIV/AIDS treatment.

This innovative treatment — which would evolve into HAART, or highly active antiretroviral therapy — prevented the HIV from replicating in the body and delayed the progression of the disease. After the announcement, stories abounded telling of people with HIV/AIDS making dramatic recoveries from illness after using the new medications. The media, scientists, health care professionals and public officials embraced HAART as a treatment for HIV/AIDS. This institutional shift re-categorized HIV/AIDS as a treatable disease. The medicalization of HIV/AIDS re-constituted the epidemic in relation to the discourses and practices of scientific medicine. Similarly, *Body Positive* described this period largely in terms of medical developments:

> The first major breakthrough in the treatment of HIV comes in 1996, with the introduction of protease inhibitors as part of antiretroviral combination therapies. Viral loads drop, t-cells rise, and death rates plummet, even as it becomes clear that the new medications cannot "eradicate" HIV from the body and thus fall short of being a cure. The drugs also prove difficult to take, cause serious side effects, and don't work for everyone. Alongside these tremendous advances, new HIV infections remain undiminished, sharply rising among women and people of color. (Body Positive, 2006)

This chapter examines this period of the epidemic by looking first at coverage of the International AIDS conference in Vancouver by people with HIV/AIDS who attended and participated in the proceedings. After more than a decade of dissatisfaction with the availability of viable treatment options, the prospect of HAART as a cure, or even as an effective medication, was met with a combination of hope and skepticism among those involved in organizing among people with HIV/AIDS. Writing about the epidemic during this period used the experiences of those living with HIV/AIDS to document the consequences of HAART, both good and bad, and to challenge the myths generated about the prospect of eradication and the "End of AIDS." I investigate three prominent themes in PWA media on the medicalization of living with HIV/AIDS. First is an engagement with the prospect of medical science effectively treating HIV/AIDS. Second is the challenge of living with the new medications and being involved in the medical management of HIV/AIDS as a treatable disease. Third is a critique of the medical/ industrial complex that emerged at this time now that there was a market for the treatment of HIV/AIDS. Medicalization posed challenges for organizers and activists with HIV/AIDS in working toward self-empowerment and community development as the epidemic became increasingly subsumed within the institutional discourses of medicine and medical industries.

Globalization, 2000-2006

The last chapter of this book explores the globalization of HIV/AIDS as it expanded in the late 1990s to become a dominant motif in understanding the epidemic. Not long after identifying the first cases of HIV/AIDS in the United States and in equatorial Africa in the early 1980s, public officials and scientists recognized the possibility of a global pandemic (Iliffe, 2007). Yet, despite this knowledge, governments and international organizations like the World Health Organization and United Nations were slow to respond sufficiently on a global level given the magnitude of the pandemic (Knight, 2008). Through the 1990s, as rates of infection in developing nations continued to climb exponentially while rates in developed nations leveled out, national and international authorities came under increased pressure from organizations like the Global Network of People with HIV/AIDS to formulate a more concerted response to the global AIDS epidemic. In 1996 the Joint United Nations Programme on HIV/AIDS (UNAIDS) was initiated to improve the global institutional response to the epidemic. By the late 1990s, it became widely acknowledged by institutional authorities that HIV/AIDS is a global crisis perpetrated by the inequities and injustices that exist between developed and developing nation states. *Body Positive* describes this growing awareness of an expanding global pandemic as follows:

If the late 1990s saw the taming of the AIDS in the developed world, they also witnessed the explosion of the epidemic in the developing world. Even as the numbers of people with HIV escalated into the tens of millions in Africa, Asia, and elsewhere, the high cost of medications meant that most people could not benefit from antiretroviral medications. From grassroots activists to the president of the United States, focus shifted to treatment access in the developing world early in the new century. (Body Positive, 2006)

The 13th International AIDS Conference in 2000 held in Durban, South Africa, served as a pivotal moment in raising awareness of HIV/AIDS as a global pandemic. Accounts of this conference are the starting point for my analysis of organizing and activism during this period of globalization. Despite the local orientation of early organizing by people HIV/AIDS, those involved built national and international networks based on the tenet that HIV/AIDS is a crisis that cuts across geographic and socio-political boundaries. In the late 1980s, international coalitions like the Global Network of People with HIV/AIDS formed to address the rapid worldwide spread of the disease and advocate for a wider global institutional response to the pandemic. The Seventh International Conference for People Living with HIV/AIDS in 1995 in Cape Town, South Africa, concentrated on human rights and community development in endemic countries. International PWA initiatives lobbied for a more concerted global response to HIV/AIDS in endemic countries. In my investigation, I trace a number of issues — treatment neglect, women with HIV/AIDS and AIDS denialism — that emerged because of the increasing globalization of the epidemic. To conclude, I identify changes in organizing and activism by people with HIV/AIDS in relation to the re-classification of HIV/AIDS as a global health crisis.

PWA Activism and Organizing in Historical Context

Since the late 1960s, health has become a significant site of political struggle in contemporary social movements. A greater awareness of the relationship between health issues and social structural inequalities around gender, sexuality, class, race and social stigma provides a common ground between the women's health movement, the independent living movement, organizing around gay and lesbian health, the community-based response to HIV/AIDS and social movements in health in general (Bayer, 1986; Sears, 1991). As Sears (1991) has noted, such community organizing arose "out of the intersection of a health crisis and the struggle against oppression" (p. 42). In each case, activists have mobilized in response to the societal neglect shown toward the civil rights and the health and social needs of marginalized or oppressed communities (Clarke, 1993; Withorn, 1980; Leonardis & Mauri, 1992; Wilkinson, & Kitzinger, 1993).

In the context of social movements in health, those most affected by health problems and social issues have been encouraged to organize in order to question and challenge the expertise exercised by health professionals and state officials. In doing so, they have demanded that health be treated not exclusively as a physiological condition, but as a social and political issue that must be addressed. Sears (1991) refers to this form of political organizing as "health from below":

> The politics of health from below often starts with concerns about the coercive aspects of state control. [It is] a struggle through which those most affected by specific health threats take power over the resources, knowledge and conditions of life necessary to procure well-being. (p. 32)

The idea of "health from below" suggests that with the threat of colonization and institutional control, women, people with disabilities, gay men and lesbians, and people with HIV/AIDS are collectively realizing the need to struggle for self-determination and control of their bodies and their lives. The objective of this book is to understand this history of activism and organizing — as an example of the principle of "health from below" put into practice — in relation to transformations in the classification of HIV/AIDS as a health crisis. Over the last twenty-five years, there have been identifiable shifts in the conceptualization of the epidemic. Initially the idea of HIV as a plague affecting stigmatized and marginal groups predominated. Later, public officials and institutional authorities recognized the epidemic as public health crisis. Once effective medications emerged, HIV/AIDS became a treatable disease. Most recently, with the growing awareness of the epidemic around the world,

HIV/AIDS is a global pandemic. Over this time, despite the different trajectories of the epidemic, HIV positive communities have continued to initiate strategies of self-empowerment and community development designed to shape what it means to be involved in the decisions that affect their lives, and to "live, survive and thrive" with HIV/AIDS.

Chapter One

MOBILIZATION, 1983-1989

During the early years of the epidemic in North America, people with HIV/AIDS initiated a political movement in order to help each other survive, challenge misperceptions about the disease, call for a greater institutional response to the epidemic, and be involved in decisions that affect their lives. Organizing among people with HIV/AIDS began in the early 1980s with gay men meeting in support groups in New York and San Francisco. In 1983 this political mobilization became "official" at the second National AIDS Forum in Denver when eleven men with AIDS wrote a series of principles that formed the basis of the People with AIDS (PWA) self-empowerment movement. The Denver Principles — as they came to be known — announced at the Forum, gave momentum and direction to people with HIV/AIDS who desired to become politically involved in a grassroots response to the epidemic. Coalitions and organizations run by and for people with HIV/AIDS providing education, support and advocacy began to emerge in many cities across North America at this time. This mobilization of people with HIV/AIDS during this initial period of the epidemic set the basis for a broad-based AIDS social movement in health that placed the empowerment of those infected as a key strategy in AIDS education, support and advocacy.

There are few records of the early PWA movement. This aspect of the community-based response to HIV/AIDS has not been examined in depth in chronicles of the epidemic, though recently there has been a move to revive the Denver Principles as a central tenet for the AIDS movement. One of the few sources of information about the early epidemic are publications (newsletters, magazines, and self-help guides) created by those involved in PWA organizations, coalitions and collectives. Early PWA organizations started their own publications as a form of outreach and education and also to document an epidemic that was often ignored or misrepresented in the mainstream media. As such, they offer a glimpse into the early development of the PWA self-empowerment movement from the perspective of those who were involved.

Drawing on material from early PWA publications, this chapter charts the contours of organizing by people with HIV/AIDS during the first decade of the epidemic. To begin, I describe the historical context in which the organizing among those infected emerged in the 1980s. Following this discussion is an analysis of self-empowerment as the central strategy for enabling people with HIV/AIDS to become involved in the decisions that affect their lives. The sites for self-empowerment that emerged during this period of the epidemic include redefining the meaning of HIV, advocating for civil rights, acquiring the means for survival, and fostering social support and community development. The chapter closes by identifying critical ways that this PWA self-empowerment contributed to the community-based and institutional response to the epidemic.

Second National AIDS Forum: The Denver Principles

The national AIDS forums were initiated by the Gay and Lesbian Task Force in the United States in 1982 when it became evident that the conservative Regan administration was unlikely to treat the epidemic as a serious health threat. The forums were held in conjunction with the National Lesbian and Gay Health Conference, the first held in 1982 in Dallas, Texas (Andriote, 1999). Shortly after the CDC acknowledged the first cases of what would become identified as AIDS, rudimentary support and education programs emerged in association with local gay and lesbian community organizations. Larry Kramer (2007), reflecting on the early history of AIDS activism, has remarked on the extent to which gay and lesbian communities were directly affected by AIDS and the institutional neglect shown toward gay men with HIV/AIDS:

So many people have forgotten, or never knew what it was like. We must never let anyone forget that no one, and I mean no one, wanted to help dying faggots. Sen. Edward Kennedy described it in 2006 as "the appalling indifference to the suffering of so many." Ronald Reagan had made it very clear that he was "irrevocably opposed" to anything to do with homosexuality. It would be seven years into his reign before he even said the word "AIDS" out loud, by which time almost every gay man in the entire world who'd had sex with another man had been exposed to the virus. During this entire time his government issued not one single health warning, not one single word of caution.

With the lack of an institutional response, it was necessary to create new community-based AIDS organizations. The Gay Men's Health Crisis formed in New York City on the east coast and the San Francisco AIDS Foundation was founded on the west coast. It is in this organizational context that people with AIDS first mobilized and became more actively involved in AIDS support, education, and advocacy. In 1982, the first organization by and for people with HIV/AIDS, the PWA Coalition of San Francisco, was formed. One of the first actions organized by the group was a candlelight march:

On May 2, 1983, the first of many candlelight marches, led and organized by people with AIDS, took place. The goal of the march was to bring attention to the plight of People With AIDS and to remember those who had died. This march was the first time PWAs marched behind a banner proclaiming what was to become the motto of the PWA self-empowerment movement: "FIGHTING FOR OUR LIVES." (Callen & Turner, 1997)

Michael Callen and Dan Turner, two PWAs who wrote about their involvement in the PWA self-empowerment movement, note that in the early 1980s small groups of people with AIDS in New York and San Francisco were meeting in support groups and expressing the need to become more involved in the decisions that affected their lives. Accounts of the PWA self-empowerment movement by Callen and Turner (1997) trace its origins to the Second National Forum on AIDS in Denver,

Colorado in 1983. Attending the National AIDS Forum, they recall, was the first opportunity for PWA self-advocacy that united people with HIV/AIDS from several large urban areas:

> The idea struck like a bolt of lightening. Until then, it simply hadn't occurred to those of us in New York who were diagnosed that we could be anything more than the passive recipients of the genuine care and concern of those who hadn't (yet) been diagnosed. As soon as the concepts of PWAs representing themselves was proposed, the idea caught on like wildfire... . (Callen & Turner, 1997)

During the conference eleven gay men living with AIDS met for first time and sketched out what would become the Denver Principles. They articulated seventeen principles that were divided into four sections: recommendations for health care professionals, recommendations for all people, recommendations for people with AIDS, and a statement outlining the rights of people with HIV/AIDS. At the closing plenary session, each member of the group read a different section from the document aloud to conference delegates. It began: "We condemn attempts to label us as "victims," a term which implies defeat, and we are only occasionally "patients," a term which implies passivity, helplessness, and dependence upon the care of others. We are People With AIDS" (Callen & Turner, 1997). The full text of the "Denver Principles" has been reprinted in Crimp's (1988) anthology, *AIDS: Cultural Analysis, Cultural Activism* (p. 148).

This declaration made to an audience of health care workers was a pivotal moment in organizing by people with HIV/AIDS. According to Ariss & Dowsett (1997), the Denver Principles became a manifesto for PWA organizing because it:

> represents the earliest discursive fixation of this concept of "self empowerment" for those with the disease. It presented a new strategy for the reorganization of the identity and collective social representation of people with AIDS. (p. 136)

The principles have been described as the "Declaration of Independence, Bill of Rights, Constitution and Magna Carta rolled into one." ("Your Brighter," 2009). In his book *Surviving AIDS*, Callen (1990) goes on to add that:

> Prior to Denver, those of us with AIDS had had no voice in the AIDS organizations that had been set up to help us. The concept of PWA self-empowerment hammered out in Denver by a group of feisty PWAs was radical in its simplicity: People with AIDS should have a say in any decision making process that will affect our lives. It was the AIDS equivalent of the principle: No taxation without representation. (p. 9)

Momentum from the Denver conference led to the formation of PWA coalitions and organizations in many cities including New York, San Francisco, Los Angeles, Washington, and Vancouver. People with AIDS ran coalitions that provided a range of education and support services. A National Association of People with AIDS, advocated for in Denver, was created soon after the conference.

The idea of self-empowerment expressed in the Denver Principles is situated in a broader set of political struggles around health that emerged in the late 1960s. A greater awareness of the relationship between health issues and social structural inequalities around gender, sexuality, class, race, and social stigma provides a link between the women's health movement, the independent living movement, organizing around gay and lesbian health, the community-based response to HIV/AIDS and social movements in health in general (Bayer, 1986; Sears, 1991). As Sears (1991) noted, such community organizing arose "out of the intersection of a health crisis and the struggle against oppression" (p. 42). Activists involved in social movements have mobilized in response to the societal neglect shown toward the civil rights and the health and social needs of marginalized or oppressed communities (Clarke, 1993; Withorn, 1980; Leonardis & Mauri, 1992; Wilkinson & Kitzinger, 1993). In doing so, they demanded that health be treated not exclusively as a physiological condition, but as a social and political issue that must be addressed. This type of political organizing around health has been referred to by Sears (1991) as "health from below":

> The politics of health from below often starts with concerns about the coercive aspects of state control. [It is] a struggle through which those most affected by specific health threats take power over the resources, knowledge and conditions of life necessary to procure well-being. (p. 32)

The idea of "health from below" suggests that with the threat of colonization and institutional control, women, people with disabilities, gay men and lesbians, and people with HIV/AIDS are collectively realizing the need to struggle for self-determination and control of their bodies and their lives.

Early PWA coalitions were an expression of this idea of health from below. People with HIV/AIDS were frustrated and angry with the way the media, government, health care system, and the general public were treating them and ignoring the severity of the AIDS epidemic. Reflecting on the beginning of the PWA movement, Richard Berkowitz (as cited in Highleyman, 2004), one of the PWAs who attended the Denver conference, wrote:

> We came to Denver as sick people and left as activists. … We marched in parades, testified before legislatures, started newsletters and hot lines, organized PWA coalitions. Against a barrage of medical reports that an AIDS diagnosis was a death sentence and media images of PWAs as disfigured monsters, we gave the most stigmatized disease of our time a human face.

The conservative political climate during the 1980s meant that governments were indifferent to HIV/AIDS because the disease was seen to only affect gay men (Sears, 1991; Rayside & Lindquist, 1992). Reflecting on the early history of the epidemic, David Salyer (2006) has written about the lack of concern bordering on denial characteristic of the U.S. government stance on HIV/AIDS in the 1980s:

During the early years, President Ronald Reagan made no public acknowledgment of AIDS — even after a Hollywood pal, charismatic film and TV star Rock Hudson, was diagnosed and died. For many Americans, Hudson's death in 1985 was their first exposure to AIDS. Then, America's extreme political right wing and the usual pack of pseudo-Christian evangelical jackals seized the opportunity to demonize gay men. Reagan advisor Pat Buchanan proclaimed, "The poor homosexuals — they have declared war against nature, and now nature is exacting an awful retribution." In the absence of any prudent, discerning national leadership on the subject, people living with HIV or AIDS were routinely divided into two categories: "innocent victims" and "people who deserve to get AIDS." Hostility towards those in the latter group was palpable. People were routinely fired from jobs, evicted from their homes and denied access to healthcare.

As Salyer mentions, there was a high level of stigma, fear, and hatred toward those HIV infected, particularly during the period when the moral panic about the epidemic was at its height. The mainstream media's coverage of the epidemic created and fueled this hysteria. As Lupton (1994) has argued, "[at] the beginning of the epidemic then, AIDS was rhetorically framed ... as a lethal, violent, enigmatic, plague like disease caused by homosexual deviance" (p. 49). In addition to shaping misperceptions of HIV/AIDS among the general public, the negative and discouraging messages conveyed in the media also contributed to sentiments of futility and hopelessness about the possibility of survival for those infected.

If institutional neglect created the circumstances that made organizing a necessity, then the practical and ideological resources that made organizing possible was drawn primarily from two sources. By the early 1980s, there was an organized gay and lesbian community in most large cities in North America (Altman, 1982; Kinsman, 1987). Activism during the 1970s led to the formation of a political ideology based on a gay liberationist critique of oppressive social institutions (Kinsman, 1987; Pawluch et al, 1994). Part of these politics included the development of local and national organizations and public spaces for gay cultural institutions such as bars, bath houses, social groups, and gay and lesbian publications (Adam, 1987; Kinsman, 1987; Patton, 1985). When the first incidents of AIDS were reported, gay men and lesbians had the organizational and ideological means to develop educational programs and outreach services for those who were most severely affected by the disease. Callen and Turner (1997), writing about the history of the PWA movement, acknowledge that:

> part of the widespread acceptance of the notion of self-empowerment must be attributed to lessons learned from the feminist and civil rights struggles. Many of the earliest and most vocal supporters of the right to self-empowerment were the lesbians and feminists among the AIDS network attendees.

PWA organizing was formed from the knowledge and expertise of gay men and lesbians gained from previous organizing and activism. Gay activists were aware of the homophobia that existed within the health care system; similarly, many lesbians (and gay men) could draw on a feminist model of organizing around health issues that emphasized self empowerment, peer support, and peer education (Dreifus, 1970).The structure and aims of early PWA organizations have been, as Kinsman (1991) writes, "informed by gay movement politics and by the feminist health movement's emphasis on empowerment" (p. 216). Early PWA organizations, like the Vancouver PWA Society, were formed by gay men and modelled after women's health collectives ("In our new," 1986).

Dissatisfaction with AIDS service organizations also set the stage for organizing among people with HIV/AIDS. People with HIV/AIDS perceived the programs available to them in the early 1980s as too bureaucratic and out of touch with the changing needs and concerns of those HIV infected and affected. Callen and Turner (1997) recalled:

> New York PWAs and PWARCS [People with AIDS Related Complex]began to express growing frustration at attending too many Gay Men's Health Crisis forums in which those of us with AIDS would sit silently in the audience and hear doctors, nurses,

lawyers, insurance experts and social workers tell us what it was like to have AIDS.

As Patton (1990) has noted, "the [PWA] movement was initially a self help movement which ran parallel to the emergent AIDS service organizations, but quickly grew into a coalition of local groups which were dissatisfied with the increasing bureaucratization of the AIDS service organizations" (p. 10). Establishing independent organizations was the most effective means of self-empowerment and self-representation. It enabled people with HIV/AIDS to educate, support, and advocate for each other on their own terms, and, to become more actively involved in the fight against AIDS.

The ideology of empowerment articulated at the AIDS forum in Denver set the foundation for the political mobilization of people with HIV/AIDS in the 1980s. Strub (2005) recently noted in his reflections on the current state of the PWA movement and the ongoing issue of ensuring that those infected need to be incorporated into leadership positions in AIDS service organizations:

The Denver Principles expressed a fundamental truth: to be successful, the fight against the epidemic must include the people who have the disease as equal partners in the battle. That model empowered our community to create a massive AIDS service delivery system, from scratch, in a remarkably short period of time under difficult circumstances. Do you remember the horrific stigma so many of us suffered during those earliest years? When those who hated and feared us sought to shame us into invisibility? To even quarantine and incarcerate us? When they would not work at our side, want us to live in their house, touch their dishes, use their towels or hold their children, it was our empowered voice that educated them. When the nation's political leadership failed to address the emerging crisis—and was content to watch us die—our collective empowerment gave us the political muscle to force change.

Under a climate of neglect, those most directly affected by HIV/AIDS organized services, engaged in civil disobedience, and started innovation programs designed to support those infected and prevent the spread of HIV/AIDS. In the years following the articulation of the Denver Principles, people with HIV/AIDS were instrumental in creating and advocating for safer sex practices as a means of prevention. People with HIV/AIDS involved in the PWA movement wrote "How to Have Sex in an Epidemic" which was one of the first attempts to articulate safer sex practices.

> It's hard to imagine a time when safer sex wasn't at the center of conversations about HIV in this country. But in 1983, when Richard Berkowitz, Michael Callen and Joseph Sonnabend, MD, wrote "How to Have Sex in an Epidemic," advocating condom use and low-risk sexual activity … .(Wortman, 2009)

Although controversial for linking the disease with promiscuity among gay men, the safer sex movement that emerged was influential in raising awareness and reducing the risk of infection. Later in the decade people with HIV/AIDS would be instrumental in the formation of ACT UP and AIDS AIDS NOW!, direct action groups dedicated to advocating for a wider institutional response to the epidemic. Sean Strub (1997) describes his involvement in the early years of ACT UP as a person with HIV/AIDS:

> Talk of quarantine was in the air. The FDA took forever to approve drugs. Researchers ran pitifully few — often unethical or repetitive — trials, with no community input. The few promising drugs were priced beyond greed. These were the outrages that pushed me, and thousands of others, to join ACT UP. It was an exciting time of my life, when I became part of this surging energy of angry, creative people determined to stop the dying. What we accomplished was nothing short of amazing. Not only did we change many horrendous AIDS policies of government, science and industry, but our actions raised the whole country's consciousness and compassion — to such an extent that now most politicians at least give lip service to our goals.

The excitement expressed about the successes of direct action groups by Strub is emblematic of a period in the epidemic in which the mobilization of those most directly affected by HIV/AIDS was predominant.

Sites for Self-Empowerment

Looking back at accounts of the early history the AIDS activism and the PWA movement there are several recurring sites for self-empowerment that provided a structure and an ongoing impetus for organizing among people with HIV/AIDS. The meaning of the term empowerment is often ambiguous and heterogeneous when used in reference to health and illness. As Gore (2002) has noted:

> the term "empowerment" has no particular meaning prior to its construction within specific discourses; that is, it is important to acknowledge that the meanings of words are always "up for grabs," that there are no essential meanings — only ascribed meanings. (p. 333)

Presupposing an essential definition of self-empowerment can lead to reifying and obscuring the efforts of people with HIV/AIDS to achieve "health from below." Alternatively I am interested in exploring the meaning of empowerment from the perspective of people with HIV/AIDS in relation to the social context during the early years of the epidemic in North America. PWA self-empowerment was put into practice when institutional discourses about the epidemic were challenged by proposing alternatives that reflected the needs and interests of people with HIV/AIDS. There were four predominant sites for self-empowerment in the writings by people living with HIV/AIDS. The first was contesting the treatment of people with HIV by asserting a PWA identity. Second was confronting HIV as a death sentence by highlighting and developing strategies for survival. Third was identifying forms of neglect and calling for greater attention to civil rights. And fourth was highlighting community organizing and arguing for an expanded institutional response to the epidemic. In each case, contesting institutional authority sought to improve social conditions for people with HIV/AIDS and create new opportunities for them to influence decisions that affect their lives.

People with AIDS (PWAs)

The meaning of a disease is often portrayed as being fixed in biology or in medical science. Yet, conditions like HIV/AIDS are social constructions; their meaning is fragmentary, open to interpretation, denunciation and transformation. As Treichler (1987) has argued:

> the very nature of AIDS is constructed through language and in particular through the discourses of medicine and science; this construction is "true" or "real" only in certain and specific ways - for example, insofar as it successfully guides research or facilitates clinical control over the illness. (p. 31)

Early in the epidemic medical and scientific constructions of AIDS were uncertain. Initially the set of symptoms and illnesses that were first identified among gay men in the early 1980s was identified as Gay Related Immune Disorder (GRID).

> Because of this early belief that somehow this new disease was connected to homosexual activity, the CDC first named the disease GRID, an acronym for Gay Related Immune Deficiency. Although this name was used only for a short period of time, being replaced by the name AIDS by August of 1982, this early stigma of a new disease fueled by the rampant homophobia of the early 1980s defined the early years of the epidemic. One early quote in *The New York Times* on July 3, 1981, by then-CDC spokesperson James Curran summed up the public perception at the time. "The best evidence against contagion," he said, "is that no cases have been reported to date outside the homosexual community or in women." (Graham, 2006)

This account of the early epidemic demonstrates how GRID, while short lived, categorized HIV/AIDS as a gay disease and misrepresented the way in which HIV spreads. Even after GRID became acquired immune deficiency syndrome (AIDS), an additional diagnosis, AIDS-related Complex, or ARC, differentiated between those who had some minor symptoms associated with AIDS but not all of the signs required for an official AIDS diagnosis. Callen and Turner (1997) recount this period of ambiguity about what it meant to have AIDS:

> It is important to remember that AIDS was not always called AIDS. In the early days, a number of names for this plague were proposed. But, in the late 1981 and early 1982, the name of choice was either GRID (Gay Related Immune Deficiency) or simply "it." One had "it." GRID and eventually AIDS were terms sloppily used to cover conditions ranging from lymphadenopathy through what is now called AIDS-Related Complex (ARC) to full blown or "frank" AIDS.

Robin Horowitz in *POZ* similarly describes the convolution of different diagnostic categories in the mid 1980s for people with HIV/AIDS:

> Early in the epidemic HIV-infected individuals fell into one of three categories: the first line was the one crossed after taking the antibody test (if you were asymptomatic you stayed at that first crossroad); the second line was signified by a low T-cell count, shingles and a bout with pneumocystis carinii pneumonia (PCP) that welcomed you to the wonderful world of AIDS-Related Complex (ARC); and the third and fateful line that nobody wanted to venture past was the world of the opportunistic infection and fewer than two hundred T-cells (an existence punctuated by fevers, Kaposi's Sarcoma [KS] lesions, Mycobacterium avium complex [MAI], Cytomegalovirus [CMV], Meningitis, and the endless list accompanying a full-blown AIDS diagnosis). (Horowitz, 1997)

The development of an HIV antibody test for the virus that leads to AIDS, as Horowitz recalls, meant that there were several different medical diagnostic meanings used to demarcate the disease (Flowers, 2001). At this time, many people who sought out medical care and received a medical diagnosis left the encounter feeling uncertain and confused.

Despite the proliferation of diagnostic categories, many people self-identified with an AIDS, ARC, or HIV diagnosis as a means for self-empowerment. As cited in the Denver Principles, people with HIV/AIDS resisted labels such as patient, victim, or pariah which were seen to strip them of their humanity; instead they insisted on being referred to as people with HIV/AIDS. This use of identity politics in the PWA movement has its basis in gay liberation ideologies. Patton (1990) has described organizing among people with AIDS as

> a hybrid between a gay liberation/identity model and the lobby/self-help model of such health-related groups as the Multiple Sclerosis Society..., which similarly create micro-cultures of diverse people sharing a common medically-related experience. (p. 10)

The declaration "We are people with AIDS" became the foundation for using a medically defined condition as the basis for creating a culture built around a common experience of illness and disease. This emergent culture helped those who identified as people with AIDS to use their experiences as the basis for rejecting and transforming the institutional meanings of the epidemic. Leading up to the Denver conference in 1983 there was a growing frustration among people with AIDS that they were being identified only in relation to narrowly defined, ethically questionable, and potentially debilitating social roles. At the conference, the decision was made to adopt "people with AIDS" as the preferred label in the Denver Principles:

> Bobbi Campbell passed along Mark Feldman's semantic proposition that we should insist on being called "people with AIDS." Mark felt passionately that we should reject the term "patient" or "victim." (Callen & Turner, 1997)

Early PWA activists recognized the semantic importance of asserting an identity that was self determined and consistent with the lived experiences of those most directly affected by the epidemic. Asserting a PWA identity was a repudiation of portrayals in the institutional discourses of medicine, the media and the state. Max Navarre articulated this point of view eloquently when writing for PWA publications like *Newsline* in the mid 1980s. In "Fighting the Victim Label" he writes:

> As a person with AIDS, I can attest to the sense of diminishment at seeing and hearing myself constantly referred to as an AIDS victim, an AIDS sufferer, and AIDS case — as anything but what I am, a person with AIDS. I am a person with a condition. I am not that condition. (1988, p. 146)

Navarre conveyed the frustration that people with AIDS felt toward their being treated as helpless, vulnerable, and hopeless in the face of this disease. Rather than stopping at frustration and dissent, PWAs such as Navarre went on to redefine and transform the victim label.

In the case of an AIDS patient, for instance, those infected critiqued the presumption that one's life could be reduced to a single disease category, that their prospects for living was only determined by the natural history of the disease, and that it was necessary to always defer to expert medical authority.

> Of course, there have always been patients who have challenged their illnesses and questioned medical authority, but never before had patients, as a group, affirmed their right to be exceptional. PWAs were saying no — no we will not be characterized as victims; no, we will not be experimented upon without our complete understanding and approval; no, we will not be medicated without explanation; no, we will not go out with a whimper. (Navarre, 1988, p. 145)

Critical studies of medical science and medical education have highlighted that health professionals are trained to privilege the imperatives of their vocation over the needs and interests of those living with disease (Freidson, 2007). Within this institutional context, people with AIDS fought to create new possibilities for self-advocacy in two ways: by turning a medical diagnosis into a social and political identity; by demanding that health care professionals change their view of and relationship with patients.

In the 1980s, mass media were also a key factor in misrepresenting people with HIV/AIDS as guilty victims of disease (Lupton, 1994). As a key source of information, newspapers, radio, and television contributed to the stigma, fear, and hatred toward those HIV infected, particularly during the period when the moral panic about the epidemic was at its height.

> In the media, everyone's a victim: of fire, of cancer, of mugging, of rape, of AIDS. In the world of reportage, no one is doing well. Victims sell newspapers. Does anyone consider the impact of this cult of the victim? Does anyone realize the power of the message, "you are helpless, there is no hope for you"? (Navarre, 1988, p. 146)

The idea of a "person with AIDS" was intended to help buffer the damaging effects of this victimization. Being a person with AIDS came to mean not thinking of oneself or being treated by others as morally suspect, futile, or powerless.

> I'm talking about the business of living, of making choices, of not being passive, helpless, dependent, the storm-tossed object of the ministrations of the kindly well. These are the pejorative connotations of victim that PWAs find unacceptable. The point is to see AIDS, when it happens to you, less as a defeat and more as an opportunity for creative life management. ... Taking the bull by the horns is a means of escaping the sentimental soap opera that the media has created around the experience of having AIDS. (Navarre, 1988, p. 145)

Community organizers and activists in the 1980s, like Navarre, who were writing about their experiences, gave voice to the efforts of people with AIDS to articulate an identity that created opportunities for self-empowerment. In 1985 Navarre wrote, "I have AIDS. Everything I do, say, believe in and live for goes against the idea of myself as a victim. I know that I am not on this earth to live out that scenario." (1985, p. 11).

Surviving and Thriving with AIDS

Sontag (1989) has written that the distinction between disease and health is deeply entrenched in the cultural values of most societies. This chasm is not benign; health signifies the positive and good whereas disease is associated with decline and decay. Sustaining the separation between the healthy and the diseased reproduces the prevailing social and moral order. When a health crisis emerges, social institutions like the media rely on the dominant cultural logics and divisions when making sense of illness and death. This frame of reference was used in media portrayals of HIV/AIDS early in the epidemic. As Crimp (1988) noted, the most notorious example is the media's use of photographs of men in the late stages of syphilis to portray gay men with HIV/AIDS. As a result, the dominant view of HIV/AIDS depicted the disease as highly contagious, not well understood, terminal, and potentially more devastating than any prior epidemic (Lupton, 1994). As Crawford (1994) has argued, such representations twinned HIV/AIDS with death and thus reinforced divisions between the healthy and the diseased. As a result, images and stories in the media about people with HIV/AIDS tended to focus on contagion and death (Bayer, 1991). Portrayals of people with HIV/AIDS stressed the inevitability of sickness and death even though it was evident early in the epidemic that many of those infected were not automatically becoming sick or dying.

The institutional framing of HIV/AIDS as a death sentence set the parameters for a second site for PWA self empowerment. Community organizing by people with HIV/AIDS in the 1980s advocated the idea of survival as a challenge to the perception of the disease as inevitably terminal. In 1987 the PWA Coalition of New York published *Surviving and Thriving with AIDS: Hints for the Newly Diagnosed*. The edited book was a compilation of poetry, advice, interviews and information by people with AIDS.

You hold in your hands the legacy of many who have come before you. It represents the collected wisdom of almost six years of struggle against a deadly, stubborn enemy: AIDS. ... As one of the lucky ones — as someone who has survived more than 4 years after my diagnosis — I have felt the need to pass along what I have learned from my own experiences and to keep alive the wisdom developed by the many "generations" of People with AIDS I have known. The brave and singular men to whom this guide is dedicated each played a unique and selfless role in proposing, developing, living and promoting the concept of PWA self-empowerment. (Callen, 1987, p. ix)

The initiative is an example of how people with HIV/AIDS used their own expertise to inform and educate those who are just learning about the disease. During this period of the epidemic, a diagnosis came with the message that AIDS was a death sentence. As expressed in the PWA coalition guide, self-empowerment meant developing strategies for survival in the face of a terminal diagnosis:

AIDS need not be viewed as a death sentence. There is life after diagnosis. We must fight to retain as much control over our lives as possible. These are the overarching principles which resonate throughout the essays collected from a diverse group of authors. Many of the authors of this collection are living those beliefs today. Others died proving the truth of these premises. (Callen, 1987, p. ix)

The stories, advice and information given in *Surviving and Thriving with AIDS* are indicative of efforts among people with AIDS to develop the means to live with the disease in the face of widespread institutional neglect. The idea of the long term survivor became a site for contesting institutional representations of the disease and for encouraging empowerment among people with HIV/AIDS. What follows are three of the most prominent strategies for survival advanced by people with HIV/AIDS during the early years of the epidemic.

Being Positive, Pragmatic, and Political. In personal accounts of living with AIDS the importance of being positive and life affirming figured prominently. With few health care options available, and the backdrop of fear and gloom about the epidemic in the media, survival meant seeking out sources of hope and optimism. One controversial resource used by many PWAs in the early 1980s was Louise Hay.

> I went to Santa Monica to a metaphysical healer named Louise Hay, who is doing some amazing work with AIDS people. I attended one of her workshops, where I met a roomful of smart, living, well informed PWAs. I left there feeling great and loving myself. ... Louise has a book called YOU CAN HEAL YOUR LIFE. Get it. Read it. And a tape you probably know about, AIDS: A POSITIVE APPROACH. Get it. Use it. (Navarre, 1985, p. 9)

Like many self-help approaches, Hay's tapes and books encouraged people to explore the linkages between mental attitude and health outcomes.

> Will Garcia and George Melton left their jobs in New York City and bought a 27 ft. Winnebago to take them around the continent to tell their story of hope and triumph over AIDS. Using a variety different disciplines — spiritual, nutritional, and conventional, these PWAs have stabilized their conditions and turned the prognosis from DEATH TO HEALTH. (Tips from long term survivors, 1989, p. 1)

Rather than dwell on the negative, people with HIV/AIDS who adopted this approach concentrated on the positive with the hope that their mindset would translate into an immune response to HIV/AIDS.

Not all people with HIV/AIDS agreed with the use of this form of positive thinking as a strategy for "healing" HIV/AIDS and advocated for a positive and aggressively pragmatic approach. In an article for the *PWA Coalition Newsline* entitled "A Good Attitude is Nice, But Won't Cure AIDS," Rob Schick wrote:

> Holding out positive thinking as a cure for AIDS that each PWA or PWArc can use here and now is even worse than selling laetrile to cancer patients. ... It is darn hard for most PWAs and PWArcs who don't deny their health status to wake each morning and cheerily sing "Oh, how wonderful I feel, as my body heals." And if cheery

> singing, learning to love oneself more a la Louise Hay, or a similar
> idea, is the trick to stopping HIV, then we do have ourselves to
> blame if we're not getting better. ... You don't have to feel guilty
> about having AIDS or ARC. (1988, p. 50)

Schick disagrees with the propensity in self-help discourses to make
people feel that they caused their illness and that if they are not getting
better it is their own fault. He alludes to another approach adopted by
people with HIV/AIDS that combines a positive outlook with a critical
pragmatism. Taking this perspective involves being open to but skeptical
about a range of modalities and explanations and relying on the knowledge
of peers and experts as key sources of information for making health care
decisions.

Descriptions of being critically pragmatic, especially later in the
decade, also included involvement in political action directed at social
injustices or PWA rights. Survival in this instance extended beyond the
personal self-empowerment to include advocating at an organizational and
institutional level.

> I started to formulate a battle plan. I was prepared to be
> confrontational. ... There were days when I felt in a fog or seemed
> to be moving under water, observing this weak little man with
> sadness and pity. Then I'd emerge for a few hours seeing everything
> crystal clear and living wide awake, each moment being now, now,
> now. Gradually my mood swings would start to even out. I became
> more politically active. In October I stood up for myself and other
> gay people by getting arrested at the Supreme Court. My body never
> felt stronger. (C., 1988, p. 9)

The extent to which people with HIV/AIDS adopted an outlook toward
their illness as a strategy for survival varied extensively across this
positive, pragmatic, and political continuum. Nonetheless, as the PWA
movement mobilized and expanded in the 1980s, those living with the
disease developed a more politicized perspective toward their illness and
their health practices.

Getting Support and Living Your Life. A concern for many people with HIV/AIDS was that they would be isolated and alone because of the stigma, sickness and fear associated with the epidemic. The seclusion from being ostracised, whether self imposed or enacted by friends, family, or loved ones was seen to be physically and emotionally detrimental to people with HIV/AIDS. To counter this, many people with HIV/AIDS formed support groups to foster social ties and build relationships. As one person with HIV/AIDS wrote:

> The support group became my career. I memorized the faces of the men and women. I replayed the stories later in the week when I told my friends about the meetings. Sharing the fear would heal me. I met people who gave me courage — people who had planned their own funerals, only to find they remained alive and healthy. I heard a man ... say he had been positive for six years and was not sick. (C., 1988, p. 9)

The PWA self-empowerment movement formed out of gay men coming together in support groups to deal with their illness and the epidemic. PWA organizations that grew out of this movement placed a priority on reaching out to those infected and building a community by creating forums for socializing and social interaction. Michael Slocum and Jim Lewis (1982) wrote a creed entitled, "You are Not Alone," for Body Positive, a PWA organization they were involved in, which reflected the desire to reach out and help those newly diagnosed, as evident in this excerpt:

> You need to know that you are not alone. ... Asking for help or reaching out for support are often considered weaknesses. Consequently, a very common response to testing HIV-positive is withdrawal. We isolate ourselves, hiding the news of our status. This can be very painful. There's no need for you to handle this by yourself, and it's probably a mistake even to try to do it. You are not the only person facing this. Learn who the others are and what they have to offer. Just hearing how someone else has adjusted to living with the virus can be enough to help you realize that life is still good, that you can still have love and laughter. And you may also be

surprised to learn that your own sharing can help others. In sharing the issues that concern us, each of our voices lends strength to the others. ... Wherever you are, you can find support, or the means to create it. It just doesn't make sense for us to face the same issues without helping each other out. We are not alone. And neither are you.

Published in the late 1980s this creed is the culmination of several prior statements intended to help those newly diagnosed. Beginning in 1986 the organization Body Positive offered a wide range of services that enabled people with HIV/AIDS to reach out to one another: dances, teahouses, workshops, orientations, parties, church services, education forums, dating services, and support groups organized around common interests (gender, sexuality, and health status).

Extending the idea of getting support, in the 1980s there was a strong sentiment that people with HIV/AIDS need not abandon key aspects of their pre-diagnosis life. With the spectre of HIV/AIDS as a death sentence circulating in popular discourses there was concern that people with HIV/AIDS would too drastically change their lives. In "You are Not Alone," Lewis and Slocum warn that

> finding out that you are infected is usually overwhelming. Even if you had suspected it for some time, learning that you are can be a very traumatic experience. Testing HIV-positive has led some people to quit their jobs, quickly write out their wills, and say goodbye to their friends and family, only to discover that they aren't sick and will probably live for many years to come. It's common to perceive these results as an immediate death sentence, but this is simply not true. (1982)

Given this concern, surviving and thriving came to mean living your life — making careful, informed decisions about how to live as a person with HIV/AIDS. Central to this idea was the importance of not giving up on relationships with friends and lovers:

You may also feel that you are now damaged in some way — that no one will want to touch you or love you or that you are less desirable because you are HIV-positive. You may feel that you will never be able to love again, that no one would want to be with you if they knew that you were HIV-positive. These feelings will pass. You are not "damaged goods." You are still a valuable person, as capable of giving and receiving love as ever. You can make your own decisions, relax, and enjoy each day. This may be a struggle and you may have to find new ways of coping with daily life, but it's worth it. (Slocum & Lewis, 1982)

In a stronger statement, David Summers echoed this view that being involved in physical, loving and sexual relationships is essential to survival.

You may be asking what right do I have, as a Person with AIDS, to be having sex—even safe sex— in public. The same right as you or anyone else has. Sure my life has changed since my diagnosis; but my dick has not fallen off. What People With AIDS need as much as any medication is body contact and compassion. Most of the People With AIDS I know have just stopped having sex. Not because of their energy levels or their lesions, but because they are afraid of rejection based on their illness. I know not everyone with AIDS is up to having sex, but for those of you who are still horny, do continue to explore your sexuality in creative and healthy ways. It's not what you can't do, it's what you can do. Life is not over at diagnosis and asserting yourself as the sexual being you once were is part of the healing process. (1987)

In *Policing Desire* Simon Watney (1987) argues that the mass media turned the epidemic into a moral panic. The target of this panic was the perception that gay sexuality, and by extension of the sexuality of people with HIV/AIDS, was out of control and need to be sanctioned. The repressive social climate about sexuality created by the media, combined with an understanding of HIV/AIDS as terminal, made adjusting to a new diagnosis difficult. A key strategy for surviving, and a key site for empowerment, was facing the barriers that prevent people with HIV/AIDS from participating in social and sexual relationships.

Being Pro-Active, Involved and Informed: The absence of an institutional response directed at mobilizing resources and enacting policies designed to assist those affected negotiate through the epidemic, led to frustration and a desire to become more involved among an emerging community of people living with HIV/AIDS.

> Please do something. Perform at the peak of our own level. If you haven't been out of bed, get out of bed for an hour. If you're out of bed, wash your own damn dishes. Don't wait for someone else to give you a reason to be alive. I believe that people die because they don't understand that they have a right to live. … Let's all just be as willing as we can to change, to go forward, to ask questions, to give answers, to be a bitch, to help someone, to love someone, to love ourselves. It's only our lives (Navarre, 1985, p. 12)

In response to this situation, people with HIV/AIDS advanced an ethic of empowerment directed at survival that entailed being pro-active, involved and informed. Bobbi Cambell, one of the first HIV positive individuals to go public, addressed the mass media in 1982 wearing a pin that said "SURVIVE." His message to other PWAs was "stay informed, be cautious but not paranoid, and be supportive" (Callen & Turner, 1997).

The availability of treatments and health care was a key contested site for PWA self-empowerment. Access to the first antiretroviral medication for HIV/AIDS, azidothymidine (AZT), began in Canada and the United States in 1987. Prior to AZT people with HIV/AIDS relied on conventional and experimental treatments in an attempt to manage the range of opportunistic infection associated with a diminished immune system. In the first volume of *Surviving and Thriving with AIDS* a section is devoted to stories and reflections on treating opportunistic infections. Michael Callen (1987) wrote about his thoughts on using prophylaxis to prevent a type of pneumonia called PCP.

I and ... my physician believe that the reason I've managed to avoid getting PCP is that almost from the beginning I have taken prophylactic medications. ...As most of you know, PCP is the number one cause of death for PWAs. Therefore, anything which has a good chance of preventing its occurrence or recurrence seems like a pretty good idea to me. I have spoken with many other PWAs who are on prophylaxis. I have also spoken to many medical authorities about the pros and cons. And I have spoken to PWAs who for whatever reason have chosen not to take prophylactic medications to prevent PCP. Though I am not, of course, a doctor, I want to recommend in the strongest possible terms that PWAs seriously consider prophylaxis. (p. 48).

Callen's approach to treatment is prototypical of the ethic used and encouraged among people with HIV/AIDS regarding their health: explore what options are available, inform yourself by consulting a range of authorities and peers, be proactive by concentrating on prevention and share what you have learned. People with HIV/AIDS also wrote about the idea of using experimental and non-conventional approaches. At the time *Surviving and Thriving* was published, for instance, many people with HIV/AIDS were trying an treatment called AL 721.

The next day I began treatment with AL 721, a potent form of lecithin which makes your cell membranes resistant to viral attacks. ... During the first week of treatment, there was no change in my condition. The three of us were planning how to deal with a corpse so far from home. But after two weeks of treatment, lo and behold! I did feel stronger. My diarrhea seemed less severe. I began to eat. During the first month I gained some weight. ... When I came back to the USA, I walked off the plane — no more wheelchair. I continued my treatment by taking a heaping tablespoon of granulated lecithin mixed with a raw egg yolk daily. During June my T/4 count continued to rise, even without the Active Lipids. My sores and skin rashes disappeared. (Callen, 1987, p. 48)

Since AL 721 was not available in the United States, access to the treatment was available only by traveling to countries where it was administered. Once word spread about the treatment, people with HIV/AIDS began to formulate an AL 721 substitute or "poor man's AL 721" that could be made at home. Discussions of home remedies were accompanied with the caution that while people may feel desperate it is valuable to consider all treatments carefully from an informed, thoughtful perspective:

> It is also important to warn all of you to think long and hard before getting involved with bizarre treatments. Of course, we are desperate and scared. All the more reason to take your time and use your reason. Many of these treatments are worthless at best, and harmful at worst. Even seemingly legitimate treatments (alpha interferon and radiation for reachable KS) have done us in. Try liquid nitrogen to reduce the KS. Don't feel sorry for the doctor because there's less money involved in treatment. See if they will treat you without payment. Again, consider carefully any treatment that someone wants to charge you for. ("HIV Man," 1987, p. 54)

The accounts of using treatments in *Surviving and Thriving*, because it was intended as a guide for the newly diagnosed, arguably represent an overly optimistic and positive account of experiences with healthcare. Accounts from other sources in 1980s show optimism and promise along with frustration and disappointment. The use of complementary medicine, for instance, was often shown to hold great promise especially in the area of prevention and health promotion.

> After two days of this regimen I was fit as a whistle and convinced of the efficacy of homeopathy. We often seem to think that everything can be cured with just medicine and this is of course a misconception. We are multi-dimensional beings and AIDS is a multi-faceted problem which must be understood and healed with a variety of methods. The mental and the emotional aspects must be dealt with as well as the physical. Diet must play a major role the healing of AIDS. (Nine, 1988, p. 34)

Accounts of the health care profession, in contrast, were far more mixed. Supportive individual physicians who were directly involved or affected by the epidemic were seen to be valuable resources and allies. And in general, medicine was portrayed as having a central role to play in an institutional response. The frustration felt by people with HIV/AIDS stemmed from the inaction and ignorance in medicine regarding the epidemic.

As for the medical community I want to break it wide open. I am not interested in the time honoured image of a doctor as omniscient authority figure. I want doubts expressed. I want sharing of information. I want an active role. Particularly since medicine is so very willing to experiment on PWAs with a new wonder drug every month. (Navarre, 1985, p. 12)

The uncertainty surrounding the efficacy of conventional medications that were, at best, considered to be experimental, combined with the feeling of being taken advantage of or discriminated against by medical authorities, made it difficult for people with HIV/AIDS to trust in the conventional health care options that were available to them. This institutional uncertainty and neglect, combined with the momentum toward change initiated in the early 1980s within affected communities, set the context for the development of survival strategies like being proactive, informed and involved that were one component of a broader ethic of empowerment articulated and practiced by people with HIV/AIDS.

Advocating for Civil Rights

In his book, *AIDS in the Mind of America*, Altman (1986) observes that what was remarkable about the epidemic was the extraordinary high level of fear given the relatively low level of risk. HIV/AIDS triggered in the public imagination deeply entrenched fears around gay sexuality and sexually transmitted diseases. As a result, the reaction to the epidemic in the media, among those not directly affected, and among institutional authorities was more often than not hostile and neglectful rather than supportive and caring. Altman (1986, pp. 60-61) cites instances of discrimination that were reported during the height of AIDS hysteria in the early 1980s: police officers and fire fighters insisting on using gloves when helping people suspected of having AIDS, babies abandoned by their parents in hospitals, health care services withheld, children excluded from schools, the mistreatment of prisoners, and people fired from their jobs without cause.

Advocating for civil rights was a site for empowerment among people with HIV/AIDS in relation to their everyday encounters and to the possibility of more widespread injustices. People with HIV/AIDS writing during the first decade documented a wide range of encounters with stigmatization and discrimination. Many expressed frustration and anger from being excluded or shunned by family and friends and neglected by social institutions because of their health status:

> Although they don't know, my brother and sister-in-law must suspect. They seemed to have turned stupid and cruel and won't let their young children visit me. For now, I'm not going to say anything about it to them, because if I do, I'll blow up. I don't believe in violence but right now I find myself hoping that somebody murders George Bush — potentially the most potent of our enemies. It's clear he and the entire administration don't give a damn. That's what angers me the most; so many people in this country don't care. (F., 1988, p. 11)

Even without the direct experience of explicit discrimination, the threat of repercussions transformed what was considered to be possible in the everyday lives of people with HIV/AIDS. The chronicles of discrimination that were written not only gave voice to the difficulties that people with HIV/AIDS had to deal with on a daily basis but also demonstrated the same triumphs of those trying to transform such situations for the benefit of themselves and others.

> When I boarded the Muni underground train at the Montgomery St. station, I noticed about five teenagers with skate boards at the back of the car. They were obviously a group of kids who knew each other, and as I located an empty seat not far from them, I heard one of them say, "what if a faggot with AIDS sits by you?" They laughed. I pondered this to myself for a few moments. It took a second or two for the impact of the words to evoke a response from my limbic (mammalian) brain. When I felt the adrenalin, I turned from my seat to face the group and said loudly, "I have AIDS and

I'm a faggot. Do any of you have a problem with it?" No one expressed one. (Mallet, 1988, p. 56)

Empowerment in the face of discrimination was expressed not exclusively with lists of experienced injustices. Alongside stories of triumph, were accounts of occasions in which family, friends or even strangers were, rather than discriminatory or afraid instead became understanding, supportive and caring.

An HIV/AIDS diagnosis, or even being suspected of infection, meant that the parameters of one's life often became constricted. There were many cases in which the rights of HIV positive individuals or those suspected of being HIV positive, were questioned or suspended. Activities that would otherwise be commonplace were suddenly made problematic when the news of a person's HIV status was disclosed. Travel, for instance, became a challenge as immigration laws in most countries would not allow entry to people with HIV/AIDS. A person writing for *Body Positive Magazine* warns,

> People with HIV disease may be harassed, detained or refused admission to Canada. ... Canada has laws requiring Immigration officers to refuse admission to people who might become dependent on their health care system. This includes people with AIDS. (HIV abroad, 1989, p. 21)

In addition to travel, services that would be considered essential were cut off: people were denied access to care and social assistance, excluded from schools and places of employment, and unable to obtain adequate housing. The sentiment running across accounts of discrimination was to not let it limit self-determination: acts of intolerance and injustice are not justified, should not be accepted or tolerated and need to be redressed through personal and political action. Empowerment, in this context, meant resisting the restrictions imposed on people as a result of their infection.

Beyond addressing the constriction of one's life that can result from discrimination, and the risk of discrimination, people with HIV/AIDS were also concerned that the panic and hysteria generated by the epidemic would be used to justify withdrawing their civil liberties. The possibility of quarantine, for instance, as a policy to manage the epidemic was seen as emblematic of the steps that institutional authorities were willing to take in limiting the freedoms of those infected in order to protect that they perceived to be the public good.

> Forty two percent of those New Yorkers [polled] by the *Daily News* want us quarantined! According to *Time* a Harvard professor is drafting model AIDS quarantine legislation. Angry parents are demonstrating in Queens to protest the admission of a child with AIDS in a classroom. Insurance companies have threatened to make AIDS an undesirable disease unless they can have access to antibody data. Massive [HIV] screening of military recruits has begun. Colorado now keeps an official list of [HIV] positive individuals. A city council in Florida has passed legislation requiring mandatory antibody testing for food handlers. (Callen, 1985, p. 10)

A number of people with HIV/AIDS wrote about the need for a more concerted and explicitly political PWA movement that would oppose policies that use an HIV positive test or an AIDS diagnosis as a means of surveillance and social control. Direct action organizations like ACT UP in the United States and AIDS ACTION NOW! in Canada gave people with HIV/AIDS a forum at arms length from the more service oriented PWA organizations to express their dissent and make demands on institutional authorities. In an account of a protest by activists at the International AIDS Conference in Washington in 1988 about the lack of government action and the growing threat of invasive mandatory testing policies, one person with HIV/AIDS wrote:

> While one thousand people circled the sidewalk in front of the White House ... Ginny Apuzzo, Michael Callen, Dixie Beckham and others sat down in the middle of Pennsylvania Avenue, directly in front of the Reagan residence, blocking traffic. ... The night before Ronny Reagan had set the tone for his administration by advocating increased mandatory testing at an AmFAR benefit. ... Emotions were running high when we marched across the street to

the White House for the "arrest ceremony." ... In two separate circling lines, we protested to the delegates and media. One placard read: "NIH You're Killing Me." ... The chants continued: "Test Drugs, Not People" and "Release the Drugs." (Licata, 1987, p. 2)

In early histories of the epidemic, organizations like ACT UP figure prominently as marking the beginning of AIDS activism (Gamson, 1989; Smith, 1990). For instance, in 1989 the journal *Radical America* featured a special issue on the AIDS movement. In the introduction, ACT UP was cited as the catalyst for the AIDS movement in North America even though AIDS organizing in the United States started as early as 1981 when the epidemic emerged. Patton (1990) has been critical of such misconceptions, noting how easily the early community-based response to HIV/AIDS can be written out of discourses about the epidemic and subsequently forgotten. Writing for *POZ Magazine*, Jane Rosett (1997) makes a similar point in her eulogy to David Summers, an early person with AIDS and activist.

Too often people mark the beginning of AIDS activism with the founding of ACT UP. But by then, a generation of PWAs had already died fighting for their lives. David Summers, whose ashes were scattered long before the 1987 march on Wall Street, was a pioneering civil-disobedience warrior. In November 1985 in New York City, the blond 33-year-old cabaret singer became the first person to be arrested defending the rights of PWAs.

Rosett draws attention to the political dimension of the early PWA self-empowerment movement. There were those in the movement who expressed ambivalence about becoming too explicitly political, opting for a course of action that emphasized self-empowerment and community development over direct action protests associated with ACT UP! and AIDS ACTION NOW! Yet, it is evident that the PWA movement helped to provide the ideological foundations for direct actions organizations, and that many of those involved in direct action were also involved in PWA coalitions and organizations. Furthermore, the direct action of ACT UP! and AIDS ACTION NOW! demonstrate the way people with HIV/AIDS took up civil rights struggles — around discrimination, neglect, and social control — as a site for self-empowerment and health from below, making the point that there needed to be a more adequate and less harmful institutional response to the epidemic.

Conclusion

In North America throughout most of the 1980s, HIV/AIDS was widely misunderstood, feared, and considered a certain death sentence. The social institutions that should have mobilized in response to the epidemic, by and large, failed those most directly affected by the disease. In its place, activists and organizers using knowledge and tools formed through involvement in gay liberation and feminist struggles created a broad network of services designed to provide support education and advocacy. In one form or another, many of the organizations that were formed during this early AIDS movement are still active in "the fight against HIV/AIDS." What makes this moment in the epidemic distinctive, and sets HIV apart from prior health scares or epidemics, is that rather than returning to a subordinate role once embraced within the public sphere, people with HIV/AIDS, expanding on the movement they created in 1980s, insisted on having an active role in the generation of knowledge and formulation of policy.

    In this chapter I have described the involvement of people with HIV/AIDS in this community-based response to the epidemic. Individuals with GRID, ARC, HIV, AIDS or any of the labels given to the disease during its fluid infancy, refused to adopt the passive and subservient role of patient or victim and mobilized to form the PWA self-empowerment movement. The political ideology of the PWA movement set out in documents like the "Denver Principles" helped to mobilize people with HIV/AIDS (Counter, 1996). People with HIV/AIDS formed local and national organizations and coalitions drawing on principles of health from below, the idea that people should be involved in decisions that effect their lives. This organizing occurred first in large urban centres like New York, San Francisco, Vancouver and Toronto and then gradually expanded to include more remote and less populated centres (Rayside & Lindquist, 1992). PWA organizations have focused on providing people with HIV/AIDS with practical support, such as financial assistance, treatment information and affordable alternative therapies, as well as on creating a supportive environment for people with HIV/AIDS to empower themselves by becoming involved in support groups and other self help programs.

Archival accounts of this initial period of mobilization reveal several key issues that were taken up by people with HIV/AIDS as sites for self-empowerment. The gay men involved in formulating the Denver Principles created a new identity — the person with AIDS or PWA — which was the basis for articulating a series of rights and obligations for those infected and affected, health care workers, and the public. People with AIDS struggled to find a way of living that moved beyond the limits of identities like victim and patient, or moral labels like innocent and guilty, that were imposed upon them by institutional authorities. The idea of surviving and thriving also served as a site for empowerment. People with HIV/AIDS refused to accept their diagnosis as a death sentence and worked collectively to garner the means to health that they needed to live with AIDS. The means to health was not limited to treatments but included resisting the isolation and stigmatization of the disease that was prevalent, and destructive, in the initial years of the epidemic. Last, advocating around the civil rights of people with HIV/AIDS was a third site for self empowerment. Documenting acts of discrimination, warning against regressive policies of surveillance, and calling for a wider institutional response to the epidemic were strategies for self-determination among many people with HIV/AIDS who became involved in direct action groups like ACT UP and AIDS ACTION NOW!

The PWA self-empowerment movement helped those infected adopt and embrace a cultural and political identity, and a sense of community, by sharing their common experiences of living with HIV and AIDS. The collective actions of HIV positive individuals made important contributions to both the community based and institutional response to the epidemic during the first decade of the health crisis. People with HIV/AIDS were instrumental in creating the idea of safe sex practices and demonstrating their significance for people infected and those at risk of infection. Political resistance to policies of surveillance and quarantine showed the inherent problems of mandatory testing and reporting, and the necessity and utility of anonymous testing and programs that offered pre and post test counselling. Last, the PWA movement greatly advanced the idea of patient self advocacy. Prior to the AIDS epidemic, social movements in health — in particular the women's health movement — encouraged forms of consciousness raising about health issues among members of marginalized communities. People with HIV/AIDS showed the extent to which this ideology could be used as the basis for developing organizations, transforming societal misconceptions, and showing how it is possible for people with an illness to take an active and meaningful role in the decisions that affect their lives.

In 2003, the National Association of People with AIDS (NAPWA) marked the 20th anniversary of the Second National AIDS Forum by renewing the organization's commitment to the Denver Principles as the founding statement of the PWA self-empowerment movement. In 2007 NAPWA started the Denver Principles Project designed to draw attention to the legacy of the declaration in fostering organizing and empowerment among people with HIV/AIDS. Early in the epidemic, the declaration guided efforts among those infected to transform the meaning of AIDS so that it was no longer perceived as terminal or invoked feelings of fear, blame, or sympathy. One of the central messages of those involved in the PWA movement was the importance of stripping AIDS of all its meanings other than simply as a disease: a condition that could be treated, that deserved attention from social institutions, and that could be ended. The Denver Principles have not only served as a central ideological foundation for the initial period of mobilization described in this chapter, they have also continued to be an anchor for the PWA self-empowerment movement, and PWA organization, over the last twenty five years.

Chapter Two

NORMALIZATION, 1989-1996

In this chapter I look at a period in the AIDS epidemic between 1989 and 1996. At the close of the 1980s, people with HIV/AIDS involved in the PWA self-empowerment movement were faced with the increasing normalization of the epidemic in North America. This process of normalization emerged as the result of several converging factors. Up until this point, social institutions had been slow to embrace HIV/AIDS as a public health problem. In the 1990s, while stigma remained a serious problem, the mass hysteria and fear characteristic of early responses to the epidemic lessened and social institutions, along with the general public, became more open to the development of formal and systematic HIV/AIDS policies. The changing epidemiology of HIV/AIDS also contributed to the normalization of the epidemic. People with HIV/AIDS were living longer, healthier lives. The idea that that HIV/AIDS should be treated as a chronic, manageable rather than terminal illness gained momentum during this period. Not only were people with HIV/AIDS living longer, the composition of the movement was also shifting. In the early 1980s the PWA self-empowerment movement was initiated and advanced primarily by gay men, many with a history of involvement in gay liberation politics. As the demographics of the epidemic became more diverse, a greater cross section of HIV infected individuals started to become involved in PWA organizing.

The publications created in the 1980s, along with numerous new periodicals created between 1989 and 1996, offer a glimpse into the way this process of normalization shaped portrayals of what it meant to "live with HIV" and the direction of PWA organizing and activism. After describing the institutional and activist response to the epidemic during this period, I trace a series of themes related to normalization that emerged from stories and portraits created by and for people living with HIV/AIDS. One predominate motif was portrayals of people with HIV/AIDS that emphasized the ordinary aspects of their lives. Ordinary in this sense is meant to "give HIV a human face" by highlighting the everyday lives of ordinary people who just happen to be HIV positive. A second theme emphasized the diversity, heterogeneity, and multiplicity among people with HIV/AIDS on the basis of a wide range of social categories: class, race, gender, ability, age, health status, and sexuality. Added to the images of gay men were portraits of a much broader range of individuals and communities infected and affected by the epidemic. The chapter concludes by describing how the PWA movement continued to advance its central goals of ensuring that those infected were able to be involved in decisions that affected their lives — the idea of health from below — by responding to the increasing normalization of HIV/AIDS. PWA organizing and activism during this period was very influential in transforming institutional discourses regarding the disease that made it more possible for people with HIV/AIDS to improve their health.

5ᵗʰ International AIDS Conference: The Montreal Manifesto

The first international AIDS conference was held in Atlanta in 1985. Approximately 2000 clinical researchers, health care professionals, and public officials attended (MacInnis, 2006). Experts took up certain topics, like the risk of heterosexual transmission and the international scale of the epidemic, with limited attention to the contribution or involvement of activists, community organizers, or people with HIV/AIDS. In an article on the significance of International AIDS conferences, MacInnis (2006) writes that in Montreal "the conference was a members-only event for the AIDS establishment, a chance for scientists to meet their peers and share research. [People with HIV/AIDS] were presented mainly as abstractions" (p. 14). The conventional scientific structure of the conference was increasingly seen as being exclusionary and ignoring the community-based efforts of those living with HIV to be involved directly in the decisions that affected their lives.

At the 5th International AIDS Conference in Montreal everything changed. More than at any prior conference, organizers made provisions for the involvement of people with HIV/AIDS. Forums and receptions were organized by PWA organizations so that HIV positive delegates from around the world could meet and share their perspectives. Representatives from PWA organizations in Canada were asked to be involved in the planning of the conference. Don DeGagne (1989), a person with HIV from Vancouver, reported on his role in the conference in the *Vancouver PWA Coalition Newsletter*:

> As you know I have been extremely busy with this conference in ensuring that PWAs have a voice, in educating people about what we live with, that we are human beings and not numbers and that we are part of solution not the problem. ... The opening ceremony presented a very well received videotaped view of Kevin Brown [a PWA activist]. Warren Jensen, a co-founder of our coalition, was also present and had a brief talk with the Prime Minister. ... Looking back I realize that we far exceeded our objectives. (p. 4)

DeGagne (1989) continues by describing meetings between PWA delegates and government officials — "I spoke to Minister of Health Perrin Beatty personally about PWA issues and the future seems to be one of more collaboration with level of government" — and his involvement with a Communications Department — "I ... fielded approximately 50 interviews a day" — that ensured the International media at the conference could hear the perspectives of people with HIV/AIDS:

> Not only did I have the honour of being the first PWA in the history of these conferences to represent International PWAs but I was also asked to co-preside the first opening plenary along with Maureen Lau, Deputy Minister of Health for Canada. I also spoke at the end of this plenary for 10 minutes speaking on behalf of PWAs worldwide. I specifically spoke about the human side of AIDS,

empowerment, the role of PWAs in the fight against AIDS, and discrimination. (p. 4)

Based on accounts like DeGagne's it is evident that people with HIV/AIDS worldwide had, for the first time, a presence at the International conference. Writing about his time in Montreal, Michael Slocum (1989b) noted that

> I felt [a sense of community] ... at the Fifth International Conference on AIDS. I was very happy there amidst thousands of people who had some form of concern about HIV. I had a sense of "my" world up there, which probably started when I met Nick Banton, who runs the Body Positive in London. It was a great pleasure to meet a lot of people with HIV from around the world. Nick and I went to a reception sponsored by the National Association of People with AIDS and there he introduced me to a tight knit group of Europeans from various AIDS service organizations. Everyone exchanged cards and promised to exchange magazines, but mostly we just talked and laughed and drank. (p. 9)

One important difference with the Montreal conference was it no longer only served as a forum for professional experts. It was now open to those infected so that they could come together and engage in dialogue and community development that reached beyond municipal, regional, and national boundaries.

Alongside the feeling of community described by Slocum was a widespread dissatisfaction and frustration among people with HIV/AIDS regarding the lack of progress in addressing the health needs of those infected worldwide. Despite a greater overall acceptance of people with HIV/AIDS, there were still restrictions placed on their ability to travel to the conference and afford the full registration fee. Slocum (1989), again in *Body Positive*, described the action taken by PWA activists to make their presence known and their voices heard by institutional authorities attending the conference:

There are those rare moments when normal events go haywire and ceremony turn into pandemonium. So it was when AIDS Action Now! of Toronto and ACT/UP New York stormed the opening ceremonies of the Fifth International Conference on AIDS in Montreal. 300 strong, they pushed their way onto escalators in the conference center, then marched onto the auditorium stage — just moments before the proceedings were to begin. Banners waving, loudly chanting, they confronted 12,000 delegates and journalists with an angry voice from the HIV community. Many of the conference participants joined in with applause and cheers. And when the chanting subsided, a single voice exclaimed from the podium, "On behalf of people living with AIDS in Canada and all across the world, WE officially open the Fifth International Conference on AIDS!" (p. 10)

Echoing the actions of those who founded the PWA self-empowerment movement at the National AIDS Forum in Denver in 1983, plans were put in place by members of ACT UP and AIDS ACTION NOW!, in partnership with Canadian and American PWA organizations, to ensure that the perspectives of people with HIV/AIDS be heard at the conference in a way that extended beyond tokenism. At the opening ceremonies Tim McCaskell of AIDS ACTION NOW! read Le Manifeste de Montreal, of the universal rights and needs of people living with HIV. Taking a similar form as the Denver Principles, its preamble sets out to clarify and specify the scope of the epidemic, needs and rights of people with HIV/AIDS, and responsibilities of institutional authorities:

HIV disease (infection with HIV with or without symptoms) is a worldwide epidemic affecting every country. People are infected, sick and struggling to stay alive. Their voices must be heard and their special needs met. This declaration sets forth the responsibilities of all peoples, governments, international bodies, multinational corporations, and health care providers to ensure the rights of all people living with HIV disease. (Miller, 1992, p. 211)

The document contained ten demands required to ensure the rights and needs of people with HIV/AIDS: (1) that HIV be treated as a chronic, manageable condition and that having access to treatments is a moral obligation of citizens and governments; (2) the recognition that HIV is not highly infectious; (3) the implementation of a code of rights protecting the humanity of people with HIV. The code included: anti-discrimination legislation; involvement in decision making; access to treatments; anonymous testing; medically appropriate housing; no restrictions on international travel; no mandatory testing; no quarantine; reproductive rights for women; attention to the unique needs of IV drug users, prisoners, and people with disabilities; language diversity; and catastrophic/immunity with regards to treatment choices; (4) a data bank for medication information; (5) recognition of placebo trials as unethical; (6) international standardization of treatment and drug approvals; (7) international education programs; (8) unique needs of women as a result of their unequal social position; (9) an international development fund to assist poorer countries; (10) recognition of poverty as a co-factor in HIV disease. The Montreal Manifesto has been reprinted in full in Miller's (1992) *Fluid Exchanges: Artists and Critics in the AIDS Crisis.*

After the Manifesto was read, and the conference officially opened, organizers had thought the protestors would leave once they had made their demands. Writing for *POZ Magazine*, Ron Goldberg (1998) recalls the actions and significance of the protesters' refusal:

> But it was only when we refused to leave the auditorium and instead parked ourselves in the VIP section that the crowd realized that our action was more than just a symbolic protest. Despite threats and rumors of a potential "international incident," we remained in our seats, alternately chanting and cheering, and giving notice that PWAs were "inside" the conference to stay. From that point on in the crisis, researchers would have to make extra room at the table for PWAs and their advocates. What we came to see, during a week of raucous street rallies and dogged challenges to "experts," is how crucial activism is to keeping that place at the table.

The declaration of the Montreal Manifesto, and the insistence by people with HIV/AIDS at the opening ceremonies to "remain at the table" as equal participants in the deliberations, set the tone for the remainder of the conference. Encounters generated by bringing together emblazoned community activists and, for the most part, unassuming professional experts, while an innovative step, led to moments of disagreement as to the most appropriate path to take in response to the epidemic. Writing for *Body Positive*, Paul Wychules (1989) noted that

> This year's International Conference on AIDS, entitled "The Scientific and Social Challenge" was a massive, crowded spectacle ... and very difficult ground on which to build greater optimism. Over and over one heard "science takes time," "research moves slowly," and "you must be patient." ... Throughout the conference the scientific and socially active met, shared and sometimes disagreed. (p. 4)

Activists were well organized and diligent. They consistently attended sessions and asked difficult and often frustrating questions regarding the slow progress in testing and releasing treatments as well as the administration's neglect of social issues.

> Protesters from ACT UP and AIDS ACTION NOW! were visible daily, from the opening ceremonies to the last. They demonstrated in favor of anonymous testing. They appeared at plenary and specialty sessions, armed with questions and challenges. They booed ... plans for mandatory reporting and contact tracing... . They demonstrated against the exclusion of lesbian concerns and the manner in which sex worker issues were addressed. They managed to steal the front page headlines of papers nearly every day, all across the world. ... They asked that placebo controlled trials be recognized as unethical when they are the only means of access to a particular treatment. (Slocum, 1989, p. 11)

During the conference, a contingent of scientists and government officials argued that it would be more productive if there were two International meetings—one for social issues and a second for clinical science. This division was widely rejected as activists and scientists came to understand the linkages between the social, political, and scientific. Randy Shilts, at the closing ceremonies, reiterated this point to delegates:

For the first time in the history of medicine we've seen a political coalition form around a health issue. This coalition has proven the most crucial ally of AIDS science. We've also seen this constituency turn to science and ask, "What are you giving back?" The answer of scientists has largely been "you have to understand how we work, it is slow." That answer is not good enough. It is no longer the job of science to understand science. It is the job of science to understand the world and what the world expects of science. ... You are not getting hundred of millions of dollars in government research grants because you look fabulous in white coats. You're getting that money because you're supposed to produce under the deadline pressure which this horrible epidemic presents. (As cited in Slocum, 1989, p. 13)

Shilts nicely expresses the tension between politically active people with HIV/AIDS and ivory tower scientists and government officials—a tension aggravated by their intertwined fates. As Wychules (1989) notes in his account of the conference:

The two worlds cannot work well when they work separately. The timetables of the laboratory must be tempered by the crisis in the streets. And those making demands in the streets and elsewhere must know where the research is headed and why. (p. 4)

Rather than the conventional structure of a conference that limits itself to science, people with HIV/AIDS broadened the agenda to include social and political issues that bear directly upon the practice of science and its relationship to macro societal structures (Hale, 1989).

The 5th International conference and the Montreal Manifesto, like the Denver Principles, has become a landmark in the development of organizing and activism among people with HIV/AIDS. It marked a change in the inter-relationship between the community-based response to HIV/AIDS — one key component of which is the PWA self-empowerment movement — and the actions of institutional authorities toward the epidemic. In his reflections on participating at the conference, Slocum (1989) sums up his views on the legacy of the conference:

> For many, Montreal will be remembered as the moment when AIDS activism became an International force, when the human face of AIDS sent a message of urgency to the ivory towers of science and government. It was very clear that this movement has come of age, and that the voices of those living with and affected by HIV/AIDS play a significant role in both public policy and speeding the progress of drug development. (p. 11)

Until the Montreal conference, the power structures of medical scientific knowledge production had successfully kept the division and interdependency between experts and activists hidden. Members of AIDS ACTION NOW! and ACT UP, by taking over the opening ceremonies and insisting on being involved in a scientific conference, successfully disrupted and called into question embedded institutional practices regarding HIV/AIDS research, in policy development, and in our understanding of the epidemic.

The ideas articulated in Montreal — the PWA movement coming of age, the desire to give HIV a human face, the importance of social issues like diversity and poverty, debates between activists and scientists, and discussions about partnerships between community organizers and government officials — point to a shift in the involvement of people with HIV/AIDS in the community-based response to the epidemic. In the 1990s the PWA movement gained momentum as more people were diagnosed, and more of the diagnoses were made earlier in the progression of the disease. Earlier in the epidemic an HIV diagnosis was often made only after the onset of opportunistic infections and/or once a person's immune system was depleted. The availability of a test for HIV antibodies, along with greater awareness from AIDS prevention campaigns, and access to support services through AIDS organizations, meant that more people were diagnosed HIV positive prior to the onset of symptoms. The significance of the 5th International conference as a transformative moment in the epidemic stemmed in part from an expanding community of politically involved people with HIV/AIDS with a desire to bring to attention a new and more diverse set of issues and concerns. Organizing and activism by people with HIV/AIDS included the push toward redefining HIV/AIDS as a chronic manageable disease (Fee & Fox, 1992).

The shift in meaning from terminal to chronic better reflected the lives of those infected and pointed to deficiencies in health services and health policy which continued to emphasize palliative and end of life care.

At this point in the epidemic, pressure from activists and the growing perception of AIDS as a public health threat, led most governments in industrialized democracies into the fight against HIV/AIDS (Kirp & Bayer, 1992). In many countries, including Canada and the United States, governments responded by supporting community-based AIDS organizations. By this time, a network of AIDS organizations was already in place, and the health care policies of most industrialized democracies had identified community health services as a cost efficient and effective means of providing support and education (Rayside & Lindquist, 1992; Sears, 1991). The nature of this institutional response meant that AIDS organizations were not replaced by government agencies or privatized programs and services. Instead, with government support, they were able to continue and expand their services.

Government support for AIDS organizing was a double edged sword for the PWA movement. Increased government resources certainly helped PWA organizations expand and improve their services and programs. This momentum transformed small coalitions run like collectives into more formalized and extensive service organizations with staff and a board of directors. Greater and more predictable funding allowed PWA organizations to improve existing services and develop new programming. This expansion also assisted, albeit often indirectly, in the formation of new collectives and organizations that reflected the diversity among people living with HIV/AIDS. In the 1990s there was a second wave of PWA organizing by women, prisoners, haemophiliacs, injection drug users, and people of colour.

The challenge expansion posed, however, was greater institutional involvement and regulation of AIDS organizing and PWA organizing. Literature on the community based response to HIV suggests that increasing government sponsorship led to a gradual formalization and depoliticization of the services and programs (Cain, 1993). This institutionalization has been noted in studies of AIDS organizing in the United States (Patton, 1990), in Canada (Cain, 1993) and in the United Kingdom (MacLachlan, 1992). This research claims that the formalization of AIDS service organizations contradicts earlier and more political forms of AIDS activism based on gay liberation politics, community development, and self-empowerment (Segal, 1989). In Canada for instance, Kinsman (1991) argues that the rhetoric of community partnership as expressed in the National AIDS Strategy means that AIDS organizations are caught between whether to serve the interests of the state and public health or people living with HIV/AIDS. State involvement at the level of consultation and guidance has meant that government agencies and bureaucracies control funding (Cain, 1993). This form of state management encourages AIDS organizations to adopt a model of service provision that contradicts the initial aims of the community-based AIDS movement (Kinsman, 1991; Rayside & Lindquist, 1992). As AIDS organizations become more like conventional voluntary health organizations, they are less able or willing to address political and social issues such as homophobia, racism, sexism, and access to treatments (Cain, 1993). While there was more opportunity for people with HIV/AIDS to become involved in AIDS service organizations in the 1990s, increasing government regulations circumscribed their role in the organization and their capacity to advance the interests of those infected. During the 1990s many AIDS organizations began to take more seriously the need for policies directed at involving people with HIV/AIDS in AIDS work in a meaningful way (Roy & Cain, 2001).

Changes in the organizational dynamics of the PWA movement in the 1990s occurred within the broader cultural context of the disease. During the first decade of the epidemic, the public profile of HIV/AIDS was ghettoized among marginalized communities: gay men, mostly, and secondarily sex trade workers, injection drug users, and immigrants or refugees. And while this understanding of the disease persists, its hold over the public imagination was progressively shaken in the late 1980s and early 1990s through changes in the way the media portrayed HIV infection. Media coverage of public disclosures by high profile celebrities — beginning with Rock Hudson and continuing through Magic Johnson — whose image contradicted the popular view of HIV/AIDS, assisted in reconfiguring the meaning of HIV as a health threat to everyone (Lupton, 1999). Accompanying this media coverage of celebrities were news stories about the lives of people with HIV/AIDS which, rather than take up the needs and interests of those infected, emphasized the risks of infection and the need for safer sex practices. Portrayals during this period continued to propagate the misconception that some people with HIV/AIDS are responsible for their infection because of immoral or irresponsible behavior while others are innocent victims of fate. Increased media coverage of HIV in the 1990s helped bring a higher public profile to those infected and to the epidemic in general. In response, people with HIV/AIDS sought to give the disease a human face by bringing into public discourse positive portrayals based on their lives.

The Lives of People with HIV/AIDS

The 5th International AIDS Conference was a significant moment in the development of PWA organizing in North America. Activists heralded in a new era of involvement in institutional practices regarding the epidemic. This engagement with institutional discourses — be it science and the constitution of knowledge, the media and its portrayal of lived experience, or the government and the provision and organization of health services — represents a struggle over how to best meet the needs and interests of people with HIV/AIDS. In print media by people with HIV/AIDS we can see efforts within the PWA movement to engage with the hegemony of normalization. To explore this engagement in more depth, I look at two prominent themes about the lives of people with HIV/AIDS that emerged in PWA publications between 1989 and 1996. The first is representations of people with HIV/AIDS as ordinary yet extraordinary. The second is portrayals designed to recognize and celebrate the diversity of HIV infected communities. Each theme constitutes a counter hegemonic project designed to struggle over and articulate the collective identity of people with HIV/AIDS.

Ordinary and Extraordinary Lives

In *Illness as Metaphor*, Susan Sontag (1989) describes the modern cultural understanding of disease as that of two kingdoms: one for the well and one for the sick. Individuals with illnesses face being set apart from what is considered normal; ostracized as different and therefore a threat to the moral order. This kind of alienation is heightened among people with highly stigmatized diseases like HIV/AIDS (Crawford, 1994). Since the 1990s, the portrayal of people with HIV/AIDS in institutional discourses like the media, while still based on constructing difference and segregation, has become less overtly stigmatized. It is largely recognized that the disease, while still life threatening, is less frighteningly contagious and deadly (Lupton, 1999). This shift in understanding opens the possibility for people with HIV/AIDS to move from the kingdom of the sick into the social realms of the well. In the 1990s the idea that people with HIV/AIDS participated in social arenas that are conventionally closed to those with terminal or highly contagious diseases became a predominant theme in PWA print media. While examples of HIV positive involvement in the ordinary social realms were wide ranging, there are two that I examine in more depth — employment and the creative arts — as they highlight the achievements of those infected along with the challenges they face in going about their everyday lives.

Employment: A common misconception early in the epidemic, which continues, is that people with HIV/AIDS are unable to participate in regular employment because they are too sick or the disease is too infectious and will place coworkers at too great a risk of infection. The experience of sickness for people with HIV/AIDS, as is the case with many health problems, is considerably wide ranging. At the later stages of infection, or when experiencing extreme side effects from medications or symptoms from opportunistic infections, regular work may be difficult and even impossible. What became evident in the late 1980s and into the 1990s was that many people with HIV/AIDS were involved in or wanted to be involved in the workforce. Writing in 1990, Slocum realized that HIV/AIDS did not limit his ability to work and that being employed was important in learning how to have a life with HIV:

When I got my HIV test results, Death visited me immediately. "I am here" it said, And I thought, "my God do I really have to die?" My own answer was a resounding "yes." So I prepared to die. I imagined that any minute I'd start coughing, and my plan was to sit still and cough to death. But I never started coughing. ... I've done some remarkable things in the course of my HIV infection. Well, at least they are remarkable to me. I've set aside whatever demon it was that kept telling me that it's inappropriate to be successful and happy with work — and with a wave of a wand this job appeared. ... Just now I'm learning to tell this virus that it can't stop me. I have my own agenda. (1990, p. 9)

Having an agenda including employment, for Slocum, came about as he realized what is and is not possible for a person living with HIV/AIDS. At this point in the epidemic, many people with HIV/AIDS who had once discounted the idea of work were looking to employment out of necessity, personal fulfillment, and empowerment.

Yet, finding employment or staying in a job as an openly HIV positive person was not easy. There were various workplace accounts from those who would not reveal their HIV status for fear of repercussions. Not disclosing at work, or disclosing selectively, was the safer option. In a profile of Tom Morgan in *POZ magazine*, who at the time was a writer for *The New York Times*, he admits not being able to disclose his status at the newspaper:

Coming out as PWA has been [a] ... long and deliberate odyssey. Morgan ... feared that revealing his HIV status would jeopardize his health benefits. Even at the *Times*, so ballyhooed for being liberal and gay friendly? "The newsroom is light years ahead of the business side" said Morgan, who two years ago left reporting for a management post. (Schoofs, 1995)

Discrimination was common in stories of the workplace, despite the trend toward HIV being more accepted. Interestingly, reports telling of individuals being prosecuted for violating the rights of people with HIV/AIDS were perhaps even more prevalent than personal stories of mistreatment at work. The "News and Notes" section of Body Positive Magazine often provided information about court cases involving workplace discrimination:

In another case settled in May a former Delta Airlines employee whose name was placed on a company list of HIV infected employees was awarded 275,000.00. The damages were based on the employee's emotional distress due to the company's keeping a list of positive employees, their invasion of his privacy and his wrongful discharge from Delta. (Anderson, 1994, p. 9)

Successes in the courtroom signified the presence of HIV positive individuals in the workplace and the continued stigma of the disease. And yet, legal victories for people with HIV/AIDS signified an institutional acknowledgement of their rights and an endorsement of their capacity to work — a sign that employment relations were changes.

Advancements made in the workplace were also portrayed through stories about employed people with HIV/AIDS who were open about their health status. Since its inception in 1994, *POZ magazine* has devoted a section of its pages to profile people with HIV/AIDS. Quite often the portrait was about, or at least included a description of, the person's occupation. An example is the profile of Ambrose Sims, an openly HIV positive and gay police officer in Miami.

When asked to describe himself, officer Ambrose Sims says, "I'm a soft man who carries a big stick." His boss, Detective Al Boza of the Miami Beach Police department says Sims is "a role model to the homosexual and African-American communities." ... Two years ago, when Sims was diagnosed HIV positive he again began the process of coming out to his colleagues on the force. He received a good deal of support and understanding. "I'm in the good health," he says, and instantly dismisses [the] assertion that [he] is "someone who belongs behind a desk." (Perez, 1996, p. 35)

Sims gained media attention in 1995 when a woman claimed that he put her life in danger when a small amount of his blood stained her clothes in an altercation. The profile applauded Sims' courage in being open about being HIV positive as he was not obliged to disclose his health status in this situation. Sims portrait was of an ordinary cop rising to the challenge of extraordinary circumstances by fighting for his job and trying to educate people about the risks of infection in the workplace.

Like police work, the kinds of work featured in magazines like *POZ* were semi-professional or professional occupations (teachers, social service workers, nurses) that involved an aspect of public service. In the early to mid 1990s, the most prominent example of this kind of portrayal was stories about openly HIV positive politicians. In one issue there were three profiles of HIV positive men who were involved in or running for public office. The first was of Tom Duane who ran for City Council in New York in 1991:

> The hardest part of his 1991 bid for City Counsel was disclosing his status to voters. At that time, only the people close to him knew. "My parents didn't want me to come out during the campaign. They wanted me to win. But I wanted other people with HIV to know that we can do anything." He became the first openly HIV positive candidate in the country to win public office. (Minnich, 1996, p. 38)

In another interview with Duane in *Body Positive* he explains further the reasons why it was important that he disclosed his HIV status while running for election:

> I was ready to tell. I thought that people had a right to know, before they decided to vote for me, about this other part of me. I thought they could know that about me. And that it would be helpful for other people with HIV to realize you could run for city council and be HIV positive, get up early, go to bed late, go the whole day. (Mars, 1994, p. 16)

Following this was a short article about Larry McKeon who was running for state representation in Illinois:

> A former policeman, he made the news when he helped apprehend a couple of assailants beating a man. But before he embarked on his successful bid for the Democratic nomination, he worried about headlines of another sort: what would voters make of his bid be elected as the state's first openly gay and HIV positive elected official? ... In the end he believes his very presence will make a difference. "Having someone sitting as a member of the State Legislature is the ability to stand up and talk to your colleagues and

say 'wait a minute, when you are talking about people living with
HIV, you're talking about me.'" (Savage, 1996, p. 38)

The last profile was of Howard Dean who ran for State Senate in Vermont
who said about his campaign: "I made a decision not to let HIV interfere
with what I wanted to do. ... Uniformly the response I got from people was
that I would be able to run for office" (Coyle, 1996, p. 40). In each profile,
HIV positive politicians are seen to be overcoming *and* embracing their
HIV status by disclosing to the public while running for office. A key
message is that in the face of ongoing (albeit decreasing) stigma the public
is willing and able to accept, endorse and elect HIV positive candidates
into positions of institutional authority.

Not all depictions of the workplace featured people with HIV/AIDS
in conventional occupations. In fact, as Michael Slocum hinted earlier,
many job opportunities available to HIV positive individuals were in
community-based AIDS organizations. There was pressure on AIDS
service organizations (as distinct from organizations by and for people
with HIV/AIDS) to resist the conventional distinction between service
provider and client and hire HIV positive candidates into staff positions.
An article in *Body Positive* describes a teenager with HIV who gets a job,
and the often blurred line between client and staff:

> My doctor sent me to a support group for young HIV positive
> women. ... About a month later, the leader of the support group
> called and asked if I'd be interesting in helping with a program for
> young people with HIV and AIDS. ... I started meeting people with
> HIV who were leading normal lives, and eventually I landed a
> paying job as a counselor in a clinic. I made a whole new set of
> friends, mostly guys with HIV. (Marsh, 1995, p. 10)

Increased funding from government (and increasingly private sector
sources) for community-based organizations created new paid staff
positions. PWA organizations were able to hire HIV positive individuals
to do the work that they were likely doing already as volunteers. Having
a paid job, going to work, and meeting people with HIV in similar

circumstances was shown to provide a sense of purpose, security, and normalcy.

Creative Arts and Culture: Involvement in the creative arts and culture — by which I mean any form of artistic or cultural production — was a prominent theme in portraying the everyday lives people with HIV/AIDS. A short list of openly HIV positive creative artists profiled in 1990s include: dancers, painters, actors, choreographers, models, graphic artists, illustrators, photographers, musicians, graffiti artists, drag queens, porn stars, television announcers, publishers, photographers, film makers, journalists, novelists, and poets. Magazines like *POZ* and *Body Positive* consistently featured articles about the artistic accomplishments of HIV positive individuals or groups on a local, national, and international level. In the February/March of 1995 issue of *POZ* there were profiles of MTV's Real World actor, Pedro Zamora, novelist David Feinberg, television and movie actor Tom Villard, comedian Steve Moore, model and dancer Thom Collins, architect and designer Frank Israel, and photographer David Seidner.

Like the theme of employment, accounts of people with HIV/AIDS in the arts note that this is a social sphere through which many people with HIV/AIDS make a living. In a story about actor Henry Menendez, Dennis Daniel (1994) writes:

> At 29, Menendez has accomplished what most performers only dream of — he has worked nonstop for years. ... And unlike most of you, aspiring performers, he had never waited tables, he had never driven a cab and he had never worried about paying rent. (p. 20)

As in the case of Menendez, a common subtext in stories about the working lives of artists was that the art world is a space that is supportive of people with HIV/AIDS.

> Menendez's HIV status became a matter of public record last November when he posed with other member of the Broadway theatrical community for a portrait in Carolyn Jones' *Living Proof.*
> ... As it turns out, everyone from his company manager to his

fellow performers has been very supportive. "As far as theatrical community goes, I don't think there has been a better place to work and be HIV positive," he says. "I couldn't imagine being in any other profession and having the support that I have from everyone. That's something that's very positive." (Daniel, 1994, p. 20)

A profile of choreographer Neil Greenberg and his project "Not about AIDS Dance" notes that artists often use their work as a safe forum through which to disclose and make sense of their HIV status.

Of course, being HIV positive and being frank about it doesn't raise too many eyebrows today. But for Greenberg the revelation is momentous. ... "This time I wanted to make it more personal, to have the reference be about the dancers on the stage ... That was my motivation for saying I was HIV positive. In a way I needed to do it, to tell myself so that I would know it, very clearly, very openly, so that I would understand that it's not something to keep a secret. ... So the process was beneficial. It helped me heal. Now that is a buzz word, but it did it. Healing is something art can do." (Kaplan, 1995, p. 34)

One reason put forward about the affinity between the arts world and HIV/AIDS is the high proportion of performers who are infected and affected by the epidemic. In a review of Jaime Martinez's work, an HIV positive dancer, Paul Harris (1995) gives a sense of toll HIV/AIDS has taken on the artistic community:

Jaime has been diagnosed with HIV for five years. Yet his positive status is just another fact about him, of the many remarkable but not necessarily the most important. His winning attitude is inspiring, especially in the dance world which has been extremely hard hit by the epidemic. "The effect of AIDS has been devastating," Jaime says. "There is not a dance company in America that has not been affected." What is unusual is that Jaime Martinez has come to accept his HIV status in such a way that dancing has become an essential part of his treatment and recovery. (p. 12)

Despite the prevalence of HIV in many artistic communities, and their efforts to raise awareness and respond to the epidemic, there were discussions of the ongoing challenges that performers faced about disclosing their health status in their work. Articles about the television and film industry noted that HIV positive actors faced significant barriers in obtaining roles if they disclosed. Moreover, disclosure often meant they were typecast in roles about the epidemic, leading some to wonder:

> [I]f Hollywood has made it safer, why do so many remain in the closet? (Natale, 1995, p. 58)

Even more than as an avenue for employment, involvement in creative arts and culture was shown to be a forum for people with HIV/AIDS to express themselves and their distinct perspective on the disease. A prime example is the article by Jameson Currier (1994), "Hugh Steers: Portrait of an Artist in the Epidemic" published in *Body Positive*:

> At the emotional heart of Steers' paintings are the issues of illness. Finding out that he was HIV positive led Steers to throw out all distractions within his work. As he mentioned in *Connoisseur* magazine, "I've tried to turn the disease into an opportunity by asking what insights it gives me into living and confronting mortality. ... Illness is such a crucial subject ... It is all part of my having to deal with having AIDS. How do I embrace this thing and make it OK or make myself able to live with it and produce and go on from there?" (p. 19)

As Steers notes, and can be seen in many accounts by people with HIV/AIDS, he felt compelled to use art as a means of making sense of his infection. Art allowed him to share his insights with others. In a similar way, reflecting on the intersection between HIV and his photography, John Dugdale (1995) writes about his desire to work through coming to terms with the blindness that resulted from his infection and how this changed his photography.

It happened here in the apartment. I got up, took my clothes off to take bath, turned the water on, and all of a sudden I felt like a freight train hit me in the side of the head. ... It was like the vertical hold on the TV went berserk. I wanted to have a show about what happened to me. I wanted to delve into my 8 X 10 camera. It's a great big Kodak Universal Number One view camera from 1912 that I've had adapted for Polaroid film (I got rid of my Pentax because I can't see through the lens any more). Six weeks before the opening, stuff started to pour out of me like a gushing fountain of ideas and the pictures almost took themselves. (p. 55)

There were many common themes in the reflections of artists living with HIV/AIDS. Of them, two were significant to the theme of the ordinary and extraordinary and the broader theme of normalization. The first is art as a venue for making sense of HIV as something that is not devastating or overwhelming but almost incidental in their everyday lives, even if that involves facing one's mortality. Dugdale (1995), for instance, writes about what it was like for him to accept his illness:

It's like scales falling off your eyes, or ripping through a shroud or taking your first strokes in a pond. There is an incredibly delightful freedom that you feel when you realize it doesn't matter if you die. It creates a bliss that I enjoy everyday of my life. (p. 56)

The second theme that emerged in many, though not all, of the accounts by and about artists was a desire to not be seen as activists. There was an agreement among commentators that artistic expression about HIV/AIDS in the 1990s had become less explicitly political.

Critics and art historians often look for trends within the art community, and earlier this year a critic writing in *The New York Times Review* noted that the AIDS inspired political and media oriented art of the 1980s has been increasingly joined by work that is now more personal and metaphorical. (Currier, 1994, p. 16)

Artists with HIV/AIDS discussing their work in publications like *POZ Magazine* and *Body Positive* reflected this trend:

Although Steers's work has become more focused and refined because of his illness, the artist does not consider himself an activist: "I did ACT UP when it started out and I went to the big HIH demonstration, but I am not good in groups. I am also not good at anger, and it's not very helpful force for me. I have to come to terms with that, and what I can do, and what I can do is my work." (Currier, 1994, p. 19)

Echoing the words of Steers, Dugdale (1995) has also said of himself:

"I have trouble reconciling the word "politicized." I don't want to be thought of as an activist. I don't feel angry. On the contrary, I feel like I've embarked on the one of the most incredible periods that I could ever have hoped for in my life" (p. 56)

Conceptualizing their art in relation to the personal and everyday rather than the political, and distancing themselves from the more politicized work of artists in the 1980s, is a result of, and a contribution to, the normalization (and depoliticizing) of the epidemic in the 1990s.

Everyday Life: An overarching theme in portrayals of HIV positive artists and workers was that they live similar lives to their HIV negative counterparts. It is in this way that the world views them as normal, to ballast the intense stigma generated in the 1980s about HIV/AIDS and continued, though arguably to a lesser degree, in the 1990s. And yet, by achieving the ordinary, people with HIV/AIDS are also shown to be extraordinary because they have overcome the challenges of living with a critical illness. This play of the ordinary as extraordinary recurs in the profiles of people with HIV/AIDS, not just in terms of involvement in work or the arts but in many areas of their everyday life. A clear example is portrayals of people with HIV/AIDS involved in sports and leisure. The move toward HIV/AIDS as a chronic, manageable condition brought with it a greater emphasis on health promotion. Publications by and for people with HIV/AIDS started to feature more information on how to improve and maintain health. Magazine covers featured high profile HIV positive athletes like Magic Johnson ("Magic realism: Survival of a superstar") and

Greg Louganis ("Learning from Louganis"). There were images of healthy, robust HIV positive athletes involved in their sport of choice advocating the importance of staying in shape, like in the article "Sport for all ... that means you: The benefits of being positively athletic":

> Jay, a 38-year-old runner, was already a runner when he was told of his positive status in July of 1991. For him, "a lot of it is in the attitude. Too often we give in to the press. The press can be detrimental to our health. When I run it is a way of emphasizing my feelings of wellness." He runs an average of 30 — 40 miles a week which will rise to 80 miles leading up to a marathon. (Harris, 1994, p. 13)

This article profiled a series of HIV positive athletes who were training for the Fourth Annual Gay Games in 1994. It balanced accolades about their athletic accomplishments with information about current research on the benefits of regular exercise for people with HIV/AIDS. Articles such as this one rely on sport as a signifier of health at the level of the ordinary (working out and getting regular exercise) and the extraordinary (people with HIV/AIDS having the physical capacity to thrive in sports at a high competitive level). The overarching message, which ties into portrayals of the ordinary and extraordinary in work and in the arts, is that people with HIV/AIDS can participate in the public sphere like those who are HIV negative. In his reflections on opportunities for people with HIV/AIDS to participate in activities once thought to be closed, Michel Slocum (1990) notes that there

> are countless others I know facing this virus, doing remarkable things. We have to acknowledge that. I know ex-hustlers who've turned into AIDS educators. I know ex-businessmen who hated their jobs and threw them away to pursue their dreams. I know women who've put down their drugs and reclaimed their families. I know a lot of people who've come to respect and love themselves MORE. (p. 9)

Stories of accomplishments at the level of the everyday are meant to quell the fears and concerns that HIV infection is a public health risk; they make the argument that such fears should not limit the opportunities of people with HIV/AIDS. By working, creating, and taking care of themselves these portrayals of HIV positive individuals show that they are valuable contributing citizens, not pariahs or public health risks, and HIV/AIDS is a chronic and manageable, rather than terminal, disease.

Daniel Fox (1992) identifies 1989-1990 as a year of transition in the politics of HIV infection in North America. One component of this change, he argues, was the growing awareness among many health care professionals and public officials that HIV should be treated as a chronic, manageable rather than terminal illness. This shift in the definition of HIV from terminal to chronic contributed to the process of normalizing the epidemic in the 1990s. Portraits of the ordinary and extraordinary were a strategy within the PWA movement to move the normalization of living with HIV in a direction that would facilitate self-empowerment and community development.

Diversity

The categorization of HIV as gay, male disease in institutional discourses early in the epidemic meant that other HIV positive communities were often neglected and silenced. In her book, *Last Served?* Cindy Patton (1994) documents how the needs and interests of women infected and affected by HIV were only recognized by health care professionals and public officials after almost a decade into the epidemic. Fox (1992) similarly notes that it was not until 1989 that policymakers recognized that the epidemic had been spreading rapidly among disadvantaged (gay and straight) ethnic minorities. In the 1990s, HIV/AIDS policies underwent a process of normalization in that more emphasis was placed on treating HIV as an infectious disease that is, while potentially a mainstream public health threat, most prevalent among a diverse range of marginalized communities (Herdt & Lindenbaum, 1992). This shift in policy orientation toward recognizing diversity resulted from the spread of HIV infection in the 1980s across social categories cobined with pressure from PWA and AIDS activists to address the needs of neglected communities infected or at risk of infection.

This issue of diversity has been central to organizing among people with HIV because to be successful the movement must create and sustain a collective identity based first on a disease category and secondly on social background and social circumstances. From early on, those involved in PWA organizing recognized the need to include the voices of all those infected. *Surviving and Thriving with AIDS*, the landmark anthology of writing by people with HIV/AIDS in the mid 1980s, included articles from the perspective of women, children, prisoners, injection drugs users, people of different faiths, African Americans, and families (Callen, 1987). Throughout the 1980s, even with the high proportion of gay men involved, a consistent effort was made in PWA publications to provide information on a regular basis that reflected the views of a diverse range of people with HIV/AIDS. The alliance across social categories was not always easy or straightforward, though. Writing for *Body Positive* in the late 1980s, one person with HIV/AIDS notes the tension within the movement regarding the complicated identity politics emerging at this point in the epidemic:

At the 6th International Conference on AIDS in San Francisco this year, a friend of mine was walking down the street with a black woman who has AIDS. They ran into an ACT-UP demonstration for women and people of color and noticed that there were very few women and people of color in the crowd. She was angry that these white gay men were presuming to speak for her. I don't blame her for feeling that way, and I wasn't there, so I can't presume to speak for her or for the activists. But I do remember wondering ... where were the women and people of color and why didn't they get out there and scream their heads off? (Lewis, 1990, p. 19)

In the late 1980s, an awareness of diversity is one reason why PWA organizing and AIDS activism advanced the interests of marginalized communities and worked toward changing public policies regarding women, people of colour, injection drug users, and other people with HIV with divergent social backgrounds. Judging by PWA publications, while there may have not been many women and people of colour demonstrating in San Francisco in 1990, the prominence of diversity intensified into the

1990s as more people from divergent social backgrounds became involved in PWA organizing in greater numbers.

Just as portraits of people with HIV/AIDS extended into a broader range of social spheres, like the work force and the arts, an increasing representation of the lives of people with HIV/AIDS from divergent social backgrounds marked the 1990s. Between 1989 and 1996 there were a wide range of different perspectives that were given voice in PWA publications. In this section I provide a series of short vignettes that describe the point of view of people with HIV/AIDS across social relations (gender, ethnicity, age) and social circumstances (drug use, hemophilia, and incarceration). The difficulty of analyzing diversity is that social categories intersect and overlap: women with HIV/AIDS, for instance, are also people of colour, of different ages, and live in a range of social circumstances. Each person brings a distinctive perspective to their infection and the epidemic. The categories that I have chosen also intersect and overlap. The predominance of one category over another reflects the way divisions among people with HIV/AIDS were organized and represented in PWA publications. Collectively the vignettes are designed to provide a glimpse into efforts within the PWA movement to sustain solidarity while giving a voice to HIV positive individuals and communities who are trying to advance their own specific interests and needs in response to being silenced, misrepresented, and mistreated.

Women: In the late 1980s publications by and for people with HIV/AIDS began to feature more information devoted specifically to women with HIV/AIDS. For instance, River Huston, an openly HIV positive woman, started writing a regular column in *POZ* magazine about sex and sexuality. Many publications started to publish a regular "Women and HIV" column. The rationale was that up to this point the challenges that women with HIV/AIDS face — reproductive rights, exclusion from medical research and clinical trials, and inadequate health care — had not been adequately addressed. An article published in *Body Positive* entitled "HIV positive women have rights too and they are often denied" by Barbara Santee (1988), for instance, writes:

To date, the plight of women has been virtually ignored in this epidemic. Only recently have we seen information about the effect of AIDS on women, although women represent the fastest growing group of people contracting the disease.

This article goes on to point out that HIV positive women are at risk of having their civil liberties denied — the right to participate in research, have access to adequate care, or give birth or care for children — because of the patriarchal structure of institutions like the health care system and the state. Writing for a column "Women and HIV" in *Living Positive* an HIV positive woman echoes this sentiment:

Women do have problems of their own, like being pregnant, bearing an infected child, and not having any clinical trials of our own for our own infections and the myth that all HIV positive females are either single mothers or HIV drug users needs to be erased. This disease has hit all categories of women... . (R., 1992, p. 26)

An increase in the infection rate and the kind of neglect that this woman identifies, symbolic in the form of stereotyping and material in the lack of adequate care, set the context for an expansion in organizing among women with HIV/AIDS in the 1990s. Organizations, like the Positive Women's Network in Canada, were formed at this time. At the International AIDS conference held in Amsterdam in 1992, representatives from PWA organizations formed the first international network of women with HIV:

On July 15th, 33 women from 30 countries around the world gathered in Holland, in a beautiful secluded forest for a three day workshop. What was so special about that? All of the women were living with HIV. I was one of them. It was the first such international gathering of women with HIV and it was undoubtedly one of the most important events of my life. It's hard to describe how special it was to be together, to share, laugh, bitch, and work out ideas with so many people who really understand what it is like to be a woman living with this virus. ... We explored the barriers and challenges to living with HIV and developed some concrete strategies to change the situation for women. ... Most importantly, each woman who participated took away a community of support, a common vision, and perhaps, a desire to reach out to women in their own countries, and help remove the barriers that isolate us from each other. (C., 1992, p.4)

This first hand account by C. in *Living Positive* points to the growing momentum of organizing among HIV positive women at the local, national, and international level. The requirements for change articulated at this meeting reflect the general concerns of HIV positive women at this point in the epidemic: increased funding for organizations by women with HIV/AIDS; realistic portrayals of HIV positive women in the media; access to treatments and health care that reflect women's health needs; funding for support services aimed at women with HIV; the right to make choices about reproduction and the care of children; research into the risk of infection among lesbians; and the inclusion of clinical markers specific to women's health in the definition of AIDS (C., 1992).

Beginning in the early 1990s, this expansion in organizing and activism among women with HIV/AIDS could be seen in the content and organization of PWA publications (Dowd, 1994). The number of regular writers and contributors who were women with HIV/AIDS also increased during this period. *Body Positive* featured a regular comic strip entitled "The Adventures of Dottie Positive" about the trial and tribulations facing an HIV positive woman living New York. Women contributed stories about the challenges they face living with HIV, like first person accounts about the decision to have a child:

One of the first thoughts when I was told I was HIV+ was that I would never have children. I told my immunologist that I was pregnant and expected him to say "you must have a termination" but he didn't. My husband and I had to make the decision. ... Emotionally, trying to decide either to terminate or continue the pregnancy was harder than coping with being diagnosed HIV positive. ... It was so hard to know where to turn, where to find information to help us make a decision, to know if we really had a

> choice. There were so many questions, and so much to consider. (Morrison, 1991, p.14)

In addition to first person accounts, publications championed initiatives like documentaries or organizational initiatives that were about and/or created by women living with HIV/AIDS. Feature articles and profiles of prominent HIV positive women involved in organizing and activism were published on a consistent basis, like a series of pieces about the republican AIDS activist Mary Fisher in 1994:

> Mary Fisher, the genteel socialite and daughter of venerable politico Max Fisher, who rocked the now infamous 1992 Republican National Convention with her eloquent calls for compassion on AIDS, talks about her life since the watershed speech, her political party, her kids and what it means to be the planet's most famous mommy with AIDS. (Dowd, 1994, p. 32)

POZ magazine in 1995 devoted an issue to "Women and AIDS" profiling "actress, lawyer and activist" Ilka Tanya Payan and featuring articles about clinical trials, housing, childcare, mother to child transmission, and how the needs of HIV positive women continued to be not sufficiently addressed (Keeley, 1995, p. 50). The issues that women face as a marginalized group in society compounds the challenges they face as people with HIV/AIDS. The forms of oppression unique to women need to be recognized in formulating a response to HIV/AIDS. In the 1990s "women with HIV" emerged as a distinct identity within the social world of HIV/AIDS. The emergence of women with HIV as a more prominent constituency in the PWA movement helped to dispel harmful myths and stereotypes and also to have their specific needs and interests addressed within the movement and by social institutions. Interestingly, attention to these female voices and life circumstances brought to light other marginalized individuals and groups living with HIV/AIDS whose needs and interests had been neglected. The issue of reproductive rights for women, for instance, led to the constitution of children with HIV/AIDS and HIV positive families as further "affected groups" within the broader HIV/AIDS community.

People of Colour: The identity politics that led to a formation of women with HIV as a distinct category extended to the intersections between ethnicity and HIV. As in the case with women, the spread of HIV among ethnic communities in North America, combined with a growing awareness of the spread of HIV infection within endemic countries, led to mobilization within ethnic communities toward addressing HIV/AIDS. By mid decade, for instance, it was evident that many African Americans were living with HIV/AIDS and that the institutional response to the epidemic was not meeting their needs:

> Our national investment in HIV prevention, research, treatment, care and housing has improved the health and quality of life of countless persons ... living with HIV/AIDS. Tragically, African Americans are not experiencing the full benefits of this investment. In 1996, for the first time in the epidemic, the number of new AIDS cases among African Americans surpassed that of whites. AIDS is still the leading cause of death among African Americans between the ages of 25-44. Moreover, African American women account for 56 percent of the cumulative female AIDS cases and African American children represent 58 percent of the cumulative pediatric AIDS cases. (Maldonado, 1999)

In early 1990s, people with HIV/AIDS devoted more attention to issues of ethnicity in their organizing. Reflecting on the 15th anniversary of Test Positive Aware Network in Chicago, Lester Davis recalls his involvement in initiating services directed specifically for people of colour:

> I remember coming to TPAN in 1995. ... Men of color were not well represented in a lot of organizations. ... There were not a lot of men of color present at the meetings, the support groups. Timothy Gates, a former program director, myself, and a couple more people had met at his home and just thought that TPAN needed a program for African American men specifically. ... It was mainly a trial type of program, and we decided the brothers needed a safe space to meet and talk about their issues. (Pickett, 2002)

A central issue at this time was the need to make ethnicity visible in the PWA movement in order to reach out to HIV positive people of colour and build a supportive, inclusive community. In the early 1990s Alice Terson (1989), an HIV positive woman of colour, wrote about her role as an outreach worker at Body Positive:

> I know they will listen to me, a Spanish person. ... So when I go out there, I need to go out there with people are Hispanic, who are of colour, because I don't want people turning away just because they look at you and don't have that little something that says, "well, let me go beyond this." ... Some black people say that the white man is the devil. I look at Body Positive, and it's all white. ... well, I think I'm here to change it, to put some colour into it. That is why I am here. (p. 9)

Publications at this time sought to give a voice to organizing among HIV positive people of colour. In the early 1990s *Body Positive* magazine ran a series of articles exploring the challenges that HIV/AIDS poses for communities of colour:

> With discrimination, inadequate health care, rampant infectious disease, malnutrition, infant mortality, teen pregnancy, drug use, illiteracy, lack of insurance, unemployment, underemployment and homelessness, AIDS was yet another burden taxing already overburdened communities. ... Blacks and Latinos were among the least prepared to handle the rise and unabated growth of HIV/AIDS in their communities. (Slocum, 1992, p. 12)

This inquiry described the inadequate institutional response to HIV in ethnic communities and identified the barriers to mounting a community response to the epidemic.

> Nationally blacks and latinos account for 42 percent of total AIDS cases. In New York City, HIV transmission is increasing fastest among people of colour, making up 60 percent of the city's total AIDS population. 84 percent of women with AIDS and 90 percent of pediatric cases are from communities of color in New York City.

These figures represent an urgent need for services, increased
visibility, education and advocacy — all of which have been slow
to materialize. Community activists say resistance has come from
several sources: the government, the white gay community and
people of colour themselves. (Slocum, 1992, p. 12)

During the period between 1989 and 1996 initiatives were started with
PWA and AIDS organizing to address the resistance to meeting the needs
of communities of colour. In the United States organizations like Body
Positive in New York and Test Positive Aware Network started programs
specific for people of colour with HIV/AIDS, including a Spanish
language magazine, *SIDAahoran*. In Canada, the Black AIDS Network,
the Multicultural HIV/AIDS Coalition, and Aboriginal organizations were
founded to provide education, advocacy, and support to communities of
colour living with HIV/AIDS. Such efforts were intended to combat social
forces like racism, homophobia, denial, and poverty that isolate and
impoverish people of colour and lead to what one Denis Levy (1998)
refers to as "one man epidemics":

In the 1990s, the second decade of AIDS, the sharing of
contaminated syringes, unsafe sex, drugs, and alcohol are spreading
HIV/AIDS among black and Latino heterosexuals. The safe sex
message and free condom distribution has not worked nearly as
effectively as it did in the white gay male community. Moreover, the
unwillingness of many black and Latino people to take an HIV test
makes for a host of potential one-man AIDS epidemics. Nobody has
a solution. But a partnership of the entire community must be
mobilized.

The accounts of PWA organizing around ethnicity highlight an
important point with regards to diversity. The history of racism and
oppression experienced by people of colour created structural barriers to
their identification with PWA organizing as an entity in itself. Many of the
efforts in the 1990s within the PWA movement aimed to create bridges
between the existing, predominately white HIV positive community and

communities of colour, rather than expecting people of colour to integrate themselves into the movement's existing structures.

Youth: At the beginning of the second decade of the epidemic it became apparent within PWA organizing that a new generation of youth was testing HIV positive and that the existing services were not fully addressing their needs. Furthermore, disadvantaged youth were identified at this time as being at greater risk of HIV infection. In the 1990s PWA publications began exploring the challenges facing youth.

> What is it about the teen years that put [youth] at such risk for HIV infection? Engaging in high-risk behaviors, such as unprotected sex accompanied by experimentation with alcohol and drugs, increases the likelihood of spreading the infection further in this age group. Although intravenous drugs account for only a small proportion of the spread of infection, the use of other drugs and alcohol can lead to impaired judgment and unsafe sexual practices. These unsafe practices exert a differential effect on the sexes. (Carbone, 1996, p. 14)

HIV positive youth became at this time a social category of identification within PWA organizing and as more young people became involved in the movement and structures emerged to encourage their own self-empowerment and community development. One of the earliest organizations by and for people with HIV/AIDS, Positive Youth Outreach, is a good example:

> In 1990, two HIV+ youth recognized the need for services that would deal with their issues and needs. Initially, they organized a 12-week support group and eventually PYO was formed. It soon grew to become an organization where members found relief from isolation, by having access to a safe place where they could meet, share, support, and challenge one another. PYO was the first, and presently one of only a few organizations in Canada with this mandate. We continue to be run by-and-for HIV-positive youth! (Positive Youth Outreach, n.d.)

Attention to HIV positive youth helped bring into the forefront the influence of age on one's experience with HIV/AIDS. PWA publications began devoting more attention to the voices of HIV positive children, as well as youth, by encouraging them to share their perspectives in their own writing or through interviews and profiles. An example is the series of accounts by HIV positive children/youth published by *Women Alive*:

> My name is Annie and I am 12 years old. My favorite subjects are History and Art. I love mystery and true crime stories. I like to play Nintendo when my foster siblings aren't around and I don't feel well. I can't remember my life before HIV and foster care. I think that's just because it would depress me too much and it probably isn't a good idea to dwell on the past. (A., 1997)

Interestingly, the emergence of children and youth as a new constituency within the HIV community drew attention to the needs and interests of older HIV positive individuals. The elderly were seen as another ignored and neglected group living with HIV/AIDS, the assumption being that the epidemic either only infected people at the beginning or middle of their life and those infected did not live to be elderly. In response, organizations like SAGE — addressing seniors with AIDS — formed to provide treatment information, offer support groups, and help individuals makes sense of "what it means to be an older PWA" (Moore, 1993, p. 7). The social category of age further expanded the range of constituents eligible to be included under the rubric of person with HIV/AIDS, further diversifying and normalizing the epidemic.

Incarceration: Up to this point diversity has been defined according to a set of ascribed though still fluid social relations: gender, ethnicity, and age. In the 1990s categories of identification among people living with HIV/AIDS also became organized around social circumstances. One important category to emerge at this time was HIV positive prisoners. PWA publications provided prisoners with information and support and gave them a forum to voice their concerns:

> I am HIV positive and in prison. ... I wish someone out there would
> tell these people that a person in my situation can't take abuse. I
> really need to speak out publicly because I am now so exhausted and
> depressed that it's not funny. ... Thanks for letting me speak my
> mind. I feel that someone should let you people know what really
> goes on in here. (R., 1992, p. 19)

PWA organizing in the 1990s tried to draw attention to the neglect and
abuses faced by people with HIV/AIDS in prison. First-person accounts
of what it is like for prisoners highlighted the problems that inmates faced.

> My name is Kimberly Morris #OB4212. I'm an inmate at SCI-
> Muncy, a maximum institution for women, in rural Pennsylvania. ...
> Since my arrival here at SCI-Muncy with a 1 to 3 year sentence, I've
> finally discovered what it means to be a woman with AIDS. We
> aren't treated as human beings but, outcasts within a prison system.
> There is no one to help us, or give us moral support. We're being
> treated like sub-human caged animals and have no one to defend us.
> We endure daily humiliation and demoralization. We are constantly
> being asked a thousand of questions by prison employees and
> inmates in order to relieve their fears about contracting this disease.
> I'm scared to death because no one in here wants to understand me
> or my disease. I believe in myself and my fight against this madness
> called AIDS. (Morris, 1994)

Initiatives were developed to provide education, support, and advocacy
within prisons, like a program in New York that sought to give people
with HIV/AIDS an alternative to serving their sentences in prison. And,
efforts were made to provide outreach so that HIV positive prisoners
might organize and provide peer support and advocacy within the prison
system.

Injection Drug Use: Because HIV/AIDS is spread through the
exchange of blood it became evident quite early in the epidemic that
injection drug users were at risk of infection. Yet, efforts to raise
awareness to prevent the spread among drug users, and support initiatives
to help HIV positive individuals who contracted the disease by sharing

drugs, emerged slowly. AIDS and PWA organizations in the 1990s
advocated the use of needle exchange programs as harm reduction
strategies to reduce the spread of HIV/AIDS. Prevention programs like "I
Am Worth ..." were launched to raise awareness about the risks of
injection drug use.

> A bold new print and television HIV prevention campaign created
> by four San Francisco social service agencies targets substance users
> and their partners with self image enhancing messages designed to
> support their ability to reduce their risk for HIV infection. "Our aim
> is to affirm injection substance users' belief in themselves and to
> demonstrably value their worth as a person capable of changing
> their behavior ... as a former substance abuser and someone living
> with HIV, I know from personal experience that heightened self
> worth gives life. ("San Francisco AIDS Foundation")

Prevention efforts like the "I Am Worth ..." campaign illustrate how
injection drug use was treated less as a mode of transmission than it was
a specific category of identification. In the early 1990s publications by and
for people living with HIV/AIDS there are few personal first person
accounts from injection drug users or profiles of organizations or
initiatives by and for HIV positive injection drug users. In the second
volume of Callen's (1987) anthology, *Surviving and Thriving with AIDS,*
there is section devoted to AIDS and IV Drug Use.

> Last night all I could do was toss and turn and reflect on my life.
> They confirmed the positive results of my prior test. I'm not asking
> why. I know why. I'm a recovering addict. ... Once again I'm faced
> with another disease that I'm powerless over. I've watched it claim
> the lives of both people I've grown to love in the fellowship who
> had begun to recover from their addiction and those I had used with
> on the streets who never had the chance to get clean. (Sky, 1987, p.
> 264)

In accounts by injection drug users the emphasis is as much on their
struggles to overcome addiction as a disease as it is facing and living with

HIV/AIDS. The two conditions were intertwined and in many cases the primary emphasis was on managing their drug use and addiction.

Hemophilia: In the 1980s people who received blood transfusions, many of them hemophiliacs, contracted HIV through the blood services. Questions were raised about the culpability of social institutions in charge of screening donated blood for viruses and harmful substances. What emerged as a result of infections through transfusions was living with hemophilia and HIV as a category of identification in PWA organizing. PWA publications regularly published articles by hemophiliacs who were HIV positive and involved in activist and community organizations:

> Having lived with hemophilia for nearly forty years, it has been only natural to make comparisons between the old curse, hemophilia, and the new: AIDS. I've frequently found myself trying to decide just why it is that most of us have had so much more trouble coping with AIDS... . AIDS is, after all, considerably more deadly and is stigmatized by its association with behaviours our society doesn't condone. But for those of us with hemophilia, I don't think that is the toughest part. The toughest part is that we face so many uncertainties and have so little control when dealing with AIDS. (James, 1990, p. 12)

This category was controversial in that people who contracted the disease through transfusions often blamed "other" people with HIV/AIDS for their infection. This blame evoked the idea that some people with HIV/AIDS were innocent while others were responsible for their infection—something that the PWA self-empowerment movement had spent a decade fighting against. As a result, accounts of living with HIV among hemophiliacs in PWA publications sought to acknowledge the distinct needs of people with hemophilia while emphasizing their commitment to PWA self-empowerment and community development. In the 1990s Henry Nicols became a prominent hemophiliac with HIV and was profiled several times in different PWA publications.

Perhaps the most astonishing unfolding of Henry Nichol's story was
of the teenager's refusal to accept his hometown's pity or their
willingness to classify him as an "innocent victim." Henry — white,
middle class, straight and just 17 years old — insisted that he not be
considered different from other people with AIDS, whether they
were gay or used drugs. (Currier, 1994, p. 10)

Henry's profile demonstrates the level of fear and stigma regarding
HIV/AIDS that remained among the straight, middle class public in the
1990s. This story showed that many hemophiliacs with HIV lived in fear
of disclosing their status for fear of recrimination. Hiding their HIV status
was a source of stress and a barrier in receiving the care and support
necessary to managing their illnesses. Henry's message, emerging out of
and echoing the PWA movement, was that people with HIV/AIDS need
to create a collective identity, despite their differences, in order to help
one another and be involved in the decisions that affect their lives.

In the 1990s divisions in the social worlds of people with HIV/AIDS
were expressed across two types of identity categories: social relations and
social circumstances. In each case, portrayals of diversity sought to give
a voice to and advance the needs of communities infected and affected by
HIV/AIDS — to build new structures to accommodate differences
between those infected. An assumption early in the PWA movement was
that the medical category of HIV or AIDS would suffice in creating a
solidarity that would bridge the differences that individuals brought to
their diagnosis and living with illness. Instead, it was evident that the
PWA identity was expanding and fragmenting across different
communities.

We know ourselves as straight or gay, black, Hispanic, Asian or
white, IVDUs, recovering IVDUs, hemophiliacs, women or men,
and much less as people with HIV, a community rich in diversity. A
community that shares more than it differs. Our community based
response to HIV has been splintered. The predominantly white gay
male community has organized. Black and Hispanic gay
communities are organizing; people with hemophilia are organizing.
Efforts have mounted in IVDU communities, in homeless

communities. All separately. In Montreal I was struck by the words of Dr. Jonathan Mann ... "Beyond anti-discrimination and tolerance, there is a higher call — to solidarity. This solidarity gives us confidence to continue to look into the face of AIDS — and know that we will not turn away." (Slocum, 1989b, p. 9)

As Slocum notes, in the 1990s the identity "person with HIV/AIDS" was accompanied, and even trumped, by other categories of identification based on social relations and social circumstances. Not everyone was comfortable with this new emphasis on diversity as they worried it might subvert organizing among people with HIV/AIDS.

What is my problem? ... I am not a prisoner with AIDS. I am not a woman with AIDS. I am not a person of colour... . I am not an IV drug user. I am not a hemophiliac. ... I want to be clear: there is nothing wrong with addressing the needs of various groups. In fact, I think it is an obligation. But I also believe that the needs of specific individuals and groups can be addressed without excluding others. Every group I mentioned above is first and foremost comprised of human beings with AIDS. (Slocum, 1989b, p. 9)

This sentiment is echoed through the 1990s as the epidemic spreads among a more diverse cross section of society and this expansion is increasingly recognized as an issue to be addressed in the AIDS movement and by public officials and health professionals. Despite the diffusion in what it means to be a person with HIV/AIDS, there was a consistent effort to construct a collective identity across the divisions created by social relations and social circumstances. This collective identity was seen to be the basis for creating solidarity among those infected and making it possible for self-empowerment and community development in order to counter the individualizing and isolating forces of greater institutional involvement in the lives of people with HIV/AIDS.

Conclusion

In the late 1980s public institutions came under pressure from activists and community organizers to initiate a wider range of HIV/AIDS policies in response to the shifting demographics of the epidemic. Government and media campaigns were launched to raise awareness among the public about their risk of infection. Policies and programs initiated to monitor and support those at risk of infection brought the lives of those infected under greater public scrutiny by institutions like the state and medicine. This expanded institutional response in the 1990s contributed to a normalization of HIV/AIDS.

Organizing among people with HIV/AIDS contributed to and struggled to shape the direction of this transformation. In this chapter I described two axes along which this struggle took place. The first was efforts to have HIV/AIDS recognized as a chronic, manageable disease. In the 1990s the idea that the ordinary lives of people with HIV/AIDS included participating in social arenas that are conventionally closed to people with terminal or highly contagious diseases became a predominant theme in PWA print media. While examples of HIV positive involvement in the ordinary social realms were wide ranging, there are two that I examine in more depth — employment and the creative arts — as they highlight the achievements of those infected along with the challenges they face in going about their everyday lives. By portraying the expansion of people with HIV/AIDS into public sphere once considered close to them, the PWA movement sought to demonstrate how the lives of those infected had changed from the first decade of the epidemic. This shift in understanding HIV/AIDS was as important as it was necessary so that policies and services could catch up with the lives of those infected. Health care services for people with HIV/AIDS, for instance, needed to include aspects of health promotion and managing illness rather than orienting solely around end of life concerns and palliative care. To adequately meet the needs of people with HIV/AIDS, programs designed to help them have employment, families, travel, sport, leisure and long term relationships needed to be initiated and supported.

A second change in the epidemic in the 1990s was the increasing diversification of HIV/AIDS across populations at risk. This diversity helped to move the epidemic from the margin into the mainstream, even though the communities infected were still marginal to the mainstream defined as middle class, white, and straight. Rather than more mainstream it may be more accurate to say that the epidemic moved more into the public sphere because of its spread across social categories of people. PWA organizing responded to this shift by creating new structures within the movement to accommodate and acknowledge the greater diversity of people with HIV/AIDS while sustaining self-empowerment and community development as a foundational basis for solidarity among those infected. The proliferation of new PWA organizations and devoted resources across different communities raised questions about the viability of the movement as people began to identify first with social categories other than their HIV diagnosis. However, the new structures that were developed in the movement assisted in raising awareness about and developing services for a wide range of communities infected and affected by HIV/AIDS.

The process of normalization that occurred within the epidemic in the 1990s was welcomed and encouraged by people with HIV/AIDS on one level. Pathways were forged so that they could participate in social worlds normally closed to people with terminal, infectious diseases. Those in the AIDS movement, along with public officials and health care workers, recognized the wide range of people living with HIV/AIDS. At the same time, however, normalcy brought with it considerable risks. The lives of people with HIV/AIDS were exposed and open to institutional control. Policies and programs initiated by institutional authorities had the potential to individualize those infected and affected and depoliticize and subvert PWA organizing initiatives under the guise of supporting them. People involved in the PWA movement were aware of the risks of normalization and they attempted not to counter it but mitigate its harmfulness:

Despite our optimism, HIV is not yet a manageable chronic disease like diabetes. No, today AIDS is still a killer for most, a disaster for all. For all that is the important idea here. That's where the debate is going astray. AIDS is a disaster striking every country, every family, every hour of everyday all the while increasing in intensity. We must not let our "leaders" minimize us, separate us or pit us against other tragic diseases. (Wychules, 1989, p. 9)

The above concerns expressed by Paul Wychules, writing for *Body Positive* in 1989, illustrate the fine balance that was required of PWA organizing in the 1990s. It was necessary to portray the lives of people with HIV/AIDS in a way that encouraged self-empowerment and community development; to show that many people with HIV/AIDS were surviving and thriving with a disease that was increasingly becoming chronic and manageable. At the same time, this move toward the mainstream also posed the threat of making the disease disappear as a crisis that required an institutional response. The concern was that after years of neglect, ironically, the moment social institutions recognized HIV/AIDS as a serious public health risk it would also be forgotten. In the 1990s the struggle over normalization within the PWA movement was portraying the capacity and diversity of people with HIV/AIDS without diminishing or misrepresenting the extent to which the epidemic continued to be a serious public health crisis.

Chapter Three

MEDICALIZATION, 1996-2000

In this chapter I investigate a period of medicalization in the AIDS epidemic that occurred between 1996 and 2000. Until the mid 1990s medications available for HIV/AIDS — AZT (Zidovudine) being the most notable along with ddI (Didanosine) and ddC (Zalcitabine) — were not very safe, effective or long term treatment options. At the International AIDS conference in Vancouver in 1996 the results from clinical trials of a new class of medications called protease inhibitors were announced. This innovative treatment — which would evolve into HAART or highly active antiretroviral therapy — was shown to prevent the HIV from replicating in the body and thereby delay the progression of the disease. After the announcement, stories abounded telling of people with HIV/AIDS making dramatic recoveries from illness after using the new medications. HAART was embraced in the media, and endorsed by scientists, health care professionals and public officials, as *the* treatment for HIV/AIDS. Andrew Sullivan, an HIV positive writer and journalist, wrote in 1996 a *New York Times Magazine* piece entitled "When Plagues End" that "the power of the newest drugs ... is such that a diagnosis of HIV infection is not just different in degree today than, say, five years ago. It is different in kind. It no longer signifies death. It merely signifies illness." Discussions turned to whether this medical advancement can be considered a cure and if we had reached the "End of AIDS." In short, HIV/AIDS was re-categorized as a treatable disease. This development brought with it the medicalization of HIV/AIDS, meaning that the epidemic was increasingly defined and understood in relation to the discourses and practices of scientific medicine.

In the later half of the 1990s publications by and for people living with HIV/AIDS responded to this emerging and expanding medicalization. After over a decade of dissatisfaction with the availability of viable treatment options, the prospect of HAART as a cure, or even as an effective medication, was met with a combination of hope and skepticism among those involved in organizing among people with HIV/AIDS. Writing about the epidemic used the experiences of those living with HIV/AIDS to document the consequences of HAART, both good and bad, and to challenge the myths generated about the prospect of eradication and the "End of AIDS." During this period, activists and people with HIV/AIDS began to make more use of the Internet, along with print publications, to voice their concerns and share experiences about the epidemic. Drawing on this material, I examine this period of the epidemic by looking first at coverage of the International AIDS conference in Vancouver by people with HIV/AIDS who attended and participated in the proceedings. This discussion sets the context for the response to medicalization among those with ties to the PWA movement. Afterward, I consider three prominent themes in PWA media that address the medicalization of living with HIV/AIDS. First is an engagement with the prospect of medical science being able to effectively treat HIV/AIDS with the availability of new medications and a better understanding of the disease. Second is the challenge of living with the new medications and being involved in the medical management of HIV/AIDS as a treatable disease. Third is a critique of the medical/industrial complex that emerged at this time, now that there was a market for the treatment of HIV/AIDS. To conclude, I discuss the challenges that faced organizing among people with HIV/AIDS in achieving their goals of self empowerment and community development as the epidemic became subsumed more within the institutional discourses of medicine and medical industries in the late 1990s.

11th International AIDS Conference

The 11th International AIDS Conference in Vancouver has become a significant moment in the epidemic because it was the epicenter for news and debates about the possibility for significant advancements in the treatment of HIV/AIDS. In reviewing the conference for *Body Positive*, Lawrence Prescott noted that

> almost 15000 participants from one hundred twenty five countries
> attended the International Conference on AIDS ... to hear the latest
> medical, scientific and public health advances in the battle against
> AIDS. This made it the largest gathering ever of medical experts,
> health care workers, persons living with HIV/AIDS, commercial
> exhibitors, and news media. (1996, p. 19.)

The meetings addressed a wide range of issues relevant to the lives of people with HIV/AIDS including ongoing efforts at prevention, organizing among sex trade workers, the expanding global epidemic, the scarcity of government funding, and the distinct needs of HIV positive women. Dorrie Millman, a woman with HIV/AIDS, opened the conference by challenging participants to question the stereotypes they hold about the disease:

> I'm here to officially open the Eleventh International Conference on
> AIDS. I know you're probably wondering why I was chosen to open
> this International conference. Well, I have AIDS. People always ask
> me how I, a grandmother from North Vancouver, British Columbia,
> could have gotten AIDS. I tell them it really doesn't matter.
> (Timour, 1999, p. 18)

Broad social and political issues regarding the epidemic — like the need for a National AIDS strategy in Canada — were raised and discussed at the conference, especially among attendees living with HIV/AIDS (Brown, 1997). The spotlight of the conference, however, was overwhelmingly on treatment advancement and more specifically the significance of protease inhibitors and combination therapy or HAART. As Prescott observed in his report:

For the first time in many years, there were high hopes that findings concerning new treatment approaches presented at this meeting, particularly with protease inhibitors, will truly have a positive impact upon the management of HIV disease. The major topic of conversation was whether or not the new combination therapies might truly eradicate HIV. (1996, p. 19)

When asked by Prescott about the significance of the new treatments, the co-chair of the conference, Dr. Julio Montaner, responded that

if anyone had asked six to twelve months ago whether HIV could be eradicated, they would have been laughed at. Today the question not only doesn't get you into trouble, it's actually worth asking. (Prescott, 1996, p. 19)

Along with the promise of more effective medications, developments in monitoring and understanding the way HIV replicates in the human body improved clinical care, and added to the level of optimism and interest in the possibility of effectively turning HIV/AIDS into a treatable disease. In his reflections on the conference, David Barr recalls that

The 1996 Vancouver conference was the Woodstock of AIDS conferences, the "eradication conference," the promise and the glory. ... Despite my reservations about the treatment hype, there was no question that this was big news — not only the treatments but also the better understanding of how the virus affects the immune system, and the use of viral load testing in clinical practice. Everything was about to change. (2003)

The change that Barr alludes to, which came to be symbolized by the Vancouver conference, was a significant move toward seeing scientific medicine as a means by which to end the epidemic. This shift in orientation was evident not only among health care professionals, public officials, and researchers but also community organizers and activists. As Barr, writing as a treatment activist and person with HIV/AIDS, notes in his account, "even my closest colleagues had jumped on the eradication train" (2003).

Announcements made at the Vancouver International AIDS Conference about the potential benefit of new treatments were quickly taken up and amplified by the many journalists who were reporting on the meeting. Stories of eradication and the possibility of a cure were quickly taken up and institutionalized through the discourses of media organizations like the *New York Times* and the *Wall Street Journal.* The scientist who made the announcement about the possibility of eradication, Dr. David Ho, was named "Man of the Year" by *TIME Magazine.* At the end of 1996, *Newsweek* published a controversial cover story with the title "The End of AIDS?" In an article reviewing major events in the 1990s, Walter Armstrong comments in *POZ Magazine* about 1996:

> *Newsweek*'s 'The End of AIDS?' cover climaxes a season of headlines featuring cocktails, hope and hype above happy-face tales of science turning a death sentence into a chronic, manageable disease. (1999)

Even though the article in *Newsweek* questioned the idea that combination therapy was a cure — part of the byline read "the plague continues" — it helped to engender and propagate an "End of AIDS" ideology. The idea that a cure was immanent if not already available became the primary institutionalized message that resulted from the conference. This message sparked widespread rumors and discussions about the prospect of an effective medical treatment for HIV/AIDS. In his book *Dry Bones Breathe*, Rofes comments that

> Early reports of the success of protease inhibitors and combination therapies led many to believe that the treatment for which we had yearned for years had arrived. ... A few dared to use the word "cure" and at least one gay newspaper's front page was emblazoned with the headline, "Activist Says AIDS Is No Longer a Killer." Rumors circulated widely insisting that doctors in Amsterdam had published reports on patients who supposedly had HIV fully eradicated from their systems. (1998, p. 3)

Lupton (1999) noted a similar trend in media coverage of people with HIV/AIDS in Australia in the 1990s toward "a discourse of hope emerging around the notion that people infected with HIV might recover from HIV/AIDS symptoms or indeed might never fall ill" (p. 51).

In the late 1990s, the predominance of an "End of AIDS" ideology had significant consequences for the direction of an institutional response to the epidemic. It is at this moment that an AIDS medical industrial complex, driven by pharmaceutical corporations, fully emerged and flourished. The availability of a viable market for the new class of medications meant that drug companies sought to become more centrally involved in treatment and care for people with HIV/AIDS. Advertisements featuring young attractive men and women involved in healthful activities like hiking became widespread in medical journals and in publications by and for people with HIV/AIDS. The U.S. Centres for Disease Control and Prevention (CDC) raised concerns about the extent to which this type of promotion gave the message that HIV/AIDS was no longer a significant health risk (U.S. Centres for Disease Control and Prevention, 2001). This image of HIV/AIDS as a treatable disease helped to legitimate the place of pharmaceutical corporations as a key arbitrator in improving the lives and prospects of people with HIV/AIDS.

A new centralized role for medicine and the medical profession in the management of HIV/AIDS emerged in the late 1990s with this perceived triumph of medical science. As a treatable, chronic disease, those infected with HIV/AIDS were expected to enroll in care as soon as possible, sustain an ongoing relationship with their health care providers, and participate in managing their illness in a way that was consistent with the recommendations of their physician (Mykhalovskiy et al., 2004). In this environment, clinical measures of health, like t-cell counts and viral load tests, took on a heightened significance as they came to represent a person's success or failure in effectively treating their illness (Selwyn and Arnold, 1998). Adherence to a medication regime became the central organizing principle around managing HIV/AIDS. The result of this increasing reliance on medicine, as Wong and Ussher note, following the work of Selwyn and Arnold, is that "the medicalization of AIDS has reduced the complexity of living with HIV and AIDS to a causal relation between disease and treatments, thus obscuring the lived experiences in which HIV infection continues to be expressed" (Wong & Ussher, 2008, p. 127).

The medicalization of HIV/AIDS influenced the orientation of government policies, as well. Discussions among public officials and community stakeholders became more organized around issues related to treatments. Ensuring access to medications and regulating costs, for instance, became a key point of contention. There was pressure to devote more resources to research and development. More attention was given to improving guidelines that governed clinical trials than the approval of new drugs. The priority in research became evaluating and setting clinical guidelines and standards of care with regards to effectiveness of medications. Commenting on this overall shift in orientation, Rosenbrock et al (2000) note that "in the course of this development medicine once again claims the power to define and shape policies and recaptures the external resources it appeared to have lost for a number of years" (p. 1616).

In the years preceding the Vancouver International Conference, AIDS activists and community organizers were engaged in a range of efforts directed at improving the quality and availability of treatments for HIV/AIDS. A general attention to improving health — in the form advancing new treatments and developing resources devoted to health promotion and chronic health management — was an emergent issue in organizing among people with HIV/AIDS in the 1990s. Epstein (1991), for instance, has shown how the political tactics by ACT UP and AIDS ACTION NOW! influenced medical scientific practices around the development and evaluation of AIDS treatments. Similarly, Kuhn (1993) has documented the efforts of PWA groups to challenge the medical establishment in the use of experimental and alternative treatments through buyers clubs and community-based research. Looking at the PWA movement in Australia, Ariss (1996) points to the role of treatment activists in lobbying the state to improve access to alternative therapies as a complement to conventional medical approaches.

Prior to 1996 many AIDS activists and people with HIV/AIDS had already acquired years of experience being involved in organizing specifically around treatments. PWA organizations and direct action groups were aware of the clinical trials being done on protease inhibitors and approached the news of their benefits with a mixture of excitement and skepticism. In preparation for the Vancouver conference, there was discussion about what message to convey at the meetings. John S. James, writing in *AIDS Treatment News*, suggested "access for all" as a common uniting theme:

> Because of the great diversity of issues people are working on, and because of the shallowness of most news media reporting, it is often hard for TV viewers and newspaper readers to understand where protesters are coming from, what our issues are. We need a theme or sound bite to communicate one central idea immediately, to the media and to other conference delegates as well, letting people know right away that we are on their side. One possible theme is "Access for All." ... Almost everything we are now planning could fit gracefully under an Access banner. (1996)

Access began as a general motif designed to be a framework for a range of issues — "access to medical care for HIV and AIDS (and other medical care as well), to information, to prevention programs, and to other services" — yet access to new treatments was highest on the agenda:

> High prices of protease inhibitors and other HIV/AIDS drugs. Exorbitant drug prices cause different problems in different countries (depending on whether there is national health care, for example), but are destructive everywhere. All price issues ultimately affect people's access to medical care. (James, 1996)

At the conference access to treatments was a central theme as activists concentrated on exposing the injustice of pricing medications beyond what most people could afford. They targeted drug companies and governments calling for medications to be made more widely available. ACT UP fronted a banner reading "GREED = Death, end the greed. Demand access to All" playing on their earlier slogan, Silence=Death:

> AIDS Profiteers Declare War! Encouraging news about the clinical benefit of protease inhibitors means nothing if people do not have access to these drugs. By pricing drugs as high as the market will

bear without opening their books to give even the slightest justification to the cost, drug companies have declared war on people with HIV throughout the world. Their profiteering ensures that these drugs will at best bankrupt government health care programs and at worst be denied to millions of people worldwide. (ACT UP New York, 1996)

During the conference AIDS activists gave out "golden urn" awards to organizations, corporations and governments who had through their greed or negligence endangered the lives of people with HIV/AIDS. The list of awardees included: the American Medical Association, Abbott Pharmaceuticals, Serono Laboratories, Hoffman La Roche, Bayer and Merck Laboratories.

The research presented at the conference suggesting that protease inhibitors and combination therapy represented a significant advancement in the treatment of HIV/AIDS was met by activists and people with HIV/AIDS with a combination of hope and skepticism. The view of Karin Timour, reporting on the conference for *Body Positive*, reflected the point of view of many activists and people with HIV/AIDS:

As the conference began, one of the big issues was: had the cure been found, and if so, what were the implications? While it seemed that the media really wanted to have big "CURE" headlines, most people with HIV, doctors and activists had a "wait-and-see" attitude. Many feel cautiously optimistic about the protease inhibitors; they want to know how long the drugs will be effective, and they realize some people won't be able to take them at all. (1999)

At the conference activists began to raise concerns about the emergence of the "End of AIDS" ideology that would be generated out of the institutional discourses resulting from the meetings. Even at the opening ceremonies, Eric Sawyer of ACT UP New York cautioned attendees about the potential dangers of understanding the new treatments as a cure or a way of eradicating the disease:

Distinguished guests, I am going to be very blunt. I'm here to sound a wake up call to everyone attending this conference. I am afraid that you all will miss the real message from this conference. I speak especially to the media, who have started the spin that the "the cure is here, let's dance." If you think the cure is here, Think Again. The cure is not here. (1996)

He continues by pointing out one of the pitfalls of medicalization: that even if there are effective treatments, institutional and structural barriers — which are overlooked when medical solutions are given to complex social problems — will prevent most people from being able to benefit from them.

> The fact that the protease - combination-drug treatments are showing a lot of promise in the blood tests of the very few who can get them, does not mean that the cure is here. Yes the preliminary results from these hugely expensive combination treatments look great. But we are a long way from a cure, even for the rich who can afford the treatments. And we are no closer to a cure for the majority of people living with AIDS on this planet than we were ten years ago. Most PWAs can't get aspirins. (Sawyer, 1996)

Another response to the "End of AIDS" ideology that emerged from the conference was the degree to which the medications will work and the short and long term effect of them on people with HIV/AIDS. Reflecting on the conference John S. James expresses this idea as follows:

> Even with access to the best care, no one knows for sure if the great improvements for some groups in 1996 will be permanent. Will deaths continue to decrease, or will 1996 be looked back on as an exception? The answer will depend greatly on what we do now — which is why the "End of AIDS" media message is so dangerously misleading. The treatments we have must be used carefully — and continued research and development not only remain essential, but have more opportunities now than ever before to save lives. (1997)

A final concern for AIDS activism and people with HIV/AIDS that became evident at this point in the epidemic was the threat of complacency and normalization that could result from an understanding of HIV/AIDS as a treatable disease. Michael Baker expresses this concern in his coverage of Louise Binder's speech at a conference on AIDS treatment activism:

> Louise Binder ... believes that the 1996 World AIDS Conference held in Vancouver — heralded as "The Cure Conference" — was actually the birth of AIDS complacency in North America. Even though [the benefit of HAART] is complicated by the toxic side effects of the drugs, most of the world breathed a collective sigh of relief, believing that the epidemic was over. But because today's HIV treatments are a reprieve and not a cure, the need for both activism and advocacy still exists. We still need new clinical trials, new drugs, expanded access to treatments (both in North America and globally), and advocacy for improvements in the social ills that feed epidemics like HIV and AIDS — poverty, homelessness, and illiteracy. (2002)

The challenge of treatment advances, as Binder pointed out, is that activists need to ensure that the difficulties of people using the medications are not ignored and that social institutions continue to address the broader determinants of health beyond medicine that are necessary for people to effectively manage their illness.

Medicalization of Living with HIV/AIDS

Scientific advancements announced at the Vancouver International AIDS Conference and amplified by the media initiated a process of medicalization which changed the landscape of the epidemic and set the tone for efforts within the PWA self empowerment movement in the late 1990s. Advancements made in medical science shifted the meaning of HIV/AIDS so that it came to be understood as a treatable disease. In publications by and for people with HIV/AIDS between 1996 and 2000 it is possible to see several predominant themes in the response to medicalization by those involved in PWA movement. First, there was an engagement with the "End of AIDS" ideology by looking at the transformative potential of using protease inhibitors and combination therapy by people with HIV/AIDS. A second theme was portrayals of the day to day challenges of using the medications and being reliant on scientific medicine in the management of illness. The third theme was a critique of the AIDS medical industrial complex in an attempt to increase accountability and access with regards to treatment and care. Overall, representations of living with HIV/AIDS became organized much more around the discourses of medical science during this period of the epidemic. Yet, there remains a critical distance that runs throughout narratives of living with HIV/AIDS as activists and those infected assess the promises made about the new treatment landscape of protease inhibitors

End of AIDS?

The legitimacy of scientific medicine is based in large part on the widespread belief that new technologies — like treatments, vaccines or diagnostic tools — will reduce or eliminate the burden of disease. Even though many of the improvements in health over the last hundred years are due as much to public health initiatives, the expectation continues that medical research will bring about cures, often in the form of a single magic bullet, for disease like cancer, diabetes and HIV/AIDS. The "End of AIDS" ideology that was generated during and after the International AIDS conference in Vancouver emerged from this belief in the transformative capacity of medical science. Public officials, health care professionals, clinical researchers, activists and people with HIV/AIDS — even if skeptical — hoped that protease inhibitors and combination therapy would drastically improve the lives of those infected and possibly eradicate the disease completely.

The Year That Changed Everything began on a cautious note. Then in the first half of 1996 came — jackpot! — Crixivan (indinavir), Norvir (ritonavir) and Viramune (nevirapine), not to mention a test for a crucial new measure called viral load. It seemed that after 15 years of sickness and death, there were finally drugs that worked. At that summer's world AIDS conference, in Vancouver, everyone from treatment activists to stock analysts were giddy over data showing near-miraculous turnarounds and undetectable viral loads. "That conference was just buzzing with optimism and hope," recalls HIVer Tim Horn, who had written POZ's first major story on the revolutionary protease drugs only a few months before. "Suddenly, we were talking with a whole new vocabulary, about how reducing viral load was the key. Even my most cynical activist friends were elated." (Staff, 2004)

People living with HIV/AIDS contributing to publications in the late 1990s engaged with the "End of AIDS" ideology prominent during this period by drawing on their own experiences and the experiences of others infected and affected by the disease. This engagement included exploring the positive and negative consequences of using protease inhibitors and combination therapy. A central concern was highlighting the complex transformations that can occur when using new medical technologies that can potentially both improve and complicate not only health but a sense of self and everyday life. Accounts of living with the new medications and medical technologies served to articulate a critique of the eradication and "End of AIDS" scenarios that were being promoted in the media and other institutional discourses.

Lazarus Syndrome: Even prior to the official announcement that results from clinical trials of protease inhibitors held promise, stories were being circulated about the remarkable improvements in people's health as a result of using the new medications. This phenomenon was often identified as the Lazarus Syndrome. An allusion to the biblical story of Lazarus, the term refers to someone who has returned to life after serious illness or even death. The typical narrative form of this story was characterized, half tongue-in-cheek, by Peter Kurth in his article "Once upon a Lazarus." He begins by describing the stereotypical pre-protease person with HIV/AIDS:

> Call me Lazarus. I thought I'd put that in writing to see how it looks, and because everywhere I go lately people are talking about "miracles." I can't open a newspaper or flip on the television without hearing about someone leaping from his deathbed and running a marathon or opening a new AIDS musical Off-Broadway.

You know the story: A year ago, David [Kevin/Michael/ Stephen/Todd] was lying exhausted on his futon, his once-muscular frame wasted away, his features pale, gaunt and covered with lesions. Sweat poured from his brow as he toyed apathetically with his two cats, Mistle and Toe, his only companions in the barren studio he's called home ever since he was diagnosed with full-blown AIDS and had to give up his job as a personal assistant to Jennifer Aniston's veterinarian. (1997)

Having established the image of a person with HIV/AIDS as close to death, he characterizes the Lazarus effect of the new medications:

Today, thanks to the lifesaving new treatments known as "AIDS cocktails," David is back at the gym, dating the man of his dreams, planning his retirement and wondering whether he should join the MCC chorus this summer on a six-week singing tour of Nepal and Bhutan. There are thousands of Davids all over the country, men who only last year were ready to throw in the towel. Scientists call this phenomenon the Lazarus Syndrome, after Lazarus of Bethany, the man Jesus raised from the dead with three simple words at the door of his tomb: "Lazarus, come out!" (1997)

The story of Lazarus was prominent in the mainstream media and publications by and for people with HIV/AIDS in the months following the announcement of protease inhibitors and combination therapy in 1996. However, the tone of this discussion shifted quickly in PWA publications to include the challenges for people with HIV/AIDS posed by improved health and renewed life prospects:

If patients who gained renewed health because of successful AIDS treatments indeed experienced "The Lazarus Syndrome," then our man Lazarus has been up and on his feet for a couple of years now. The euphoria of his good fortune has begun to wear off a bit, and reality has set in. (King, 1999)

People with HIV/AIDS who had experienced an improvement in health began to describe the difficulties they encountered trying to reorganize their lives after having lived for many years with the understanding that they would die sooner than later from their illness.

> Life and AIDS is complex. But as much as we would like our communities to understand the details, the vast majority of AIDS messages received by those we are trying to protect are embodied in sound bites on the evening news. And the sound bites of the late 1990s have been "People with AIDS are living longer." "Lazarus back from the dead." "Back to work." "Gym memberships." "Lots of pills, but the patient looks great!" The truth, of course, is a blend of confusing public benefits, insecurity about returning to work, relationships adrift, a dangerous and unsure sexual landscape, the departure of committed advocates, and an uninformed public convinced the crisis has eased. The only certainty that remains is how creative AIDS can be in its cruelty. (King, 1999)

In this piece, Mark S. King warns that life in "the protease era" while creating new opportunities for many people with HIV/AIDS also creates new dilemmas. As he notes, people with HIV/AIDS were faced with the expectation of returning to work, paying debts, managing an often difficult medication regime, and negotiating the view, propagated in the media and often held by family, friends and acquaintance, that you are cured and the epidemic is over. In a review of highlights from 1997, staff writers at *POZ Magazine* characterized this situation succinctly:

> POZ looked at newly "healthy" HIVers pressured by their insurance companies to ditch disability and go back to work—but who were often debilitated by meds-related fatigue or diarrhea, not to mention fear that their luck wouldn't hold out. And many Lazari awoke to a financial nightmare. Remembering his dramatic mid-'90s revival, POZ contributing editor Dick Scanlan says: "I was 35 years old, with $29,000 of credit card debt—not much less than my annual income. I had to suddenly grow up, make up for lost time and organize my life. The pain of [acknowledging that] was unbelievable." (Staff, 2004)

Another complication that arose from the Lazarus syndrome was its reversal as people with HIV/AIDS who had taken the new medications but then developed resistance saw their health decline as quickly as it had returned. The realities of returning from the grave offered by people with HIV/AIDS served as a cautionary tale about the benefits of the new medications. It also critiqued the "End of AIDS" ideology, pointing out how the media, public officials and scientists had exaggerated the transformative benefits of protease inhibitors and combination therapy. As Peter Kurth concludes, "If my own experience means anything, Lazarus himself must sometimes have felt he was better off moldering in the grave ... Resurrection isn't all it's cracked up to be" (1997).

Eradication and Viral Load: Advancements in medical science in the mid 1990s included a better understanding of how HIV replicates in the human body. One of the announcements made at the International AIDS Conference in Vancouver was the possibility of eradicating HIV from the body with the use protease inhibitors and combination therapy.

> At 1996's world AIDS confab, in Vancouver, David Ho, MD, announced that his team at Aaron Diamond AIDS Research Center had likely "completely shut off viral replication" in their patients on protease therapy—and that their few remaining infected cells would "turn over and die, thus presenting the possibility that HIV will be completely eradicated." Sounds like the Cure, right? Amidst much hope and media hype, Ho was named *Time's* Man of the Year. (Staff, 2004)

It was not long after the Vancouver conference that scientists, activists and people with HIV/AIDS began to seriously question the possibility of eradication. In 1997 the treatment publication *TAGline* published an article entitled, "The Twilight of Eradication" that reported on research that showed protease inhibitors could not completely eliminate the replication of HIV:

> ... we can no longer expect the current therapeutic approaches by themselves to lead to HIV's eradication — which is really just a

fancy word for cure. ... No one should begin antiretroviral therapy with the belief that triple (or even quadruple) antiretroviral therapy is likely to eradicate HIV infection. The best we can hope for, at this time, is chronic suppression of HIV and thereby preventing disease progression, protecting the immune system from further damage, and avoiding the development of drug resistant HIV strains. (Staff, 1997)

News that protease inhibitors and combination therapy could not eliminate HIV from the body was a disappointing but not altogether unexpected revelation. Many people with HIV/AIDS using the medications were not experiencing the dramatic increases in well being. HIV positive writers, like Sidney Morris, drew on their own experiences to question the benefits of combination therapy. In an article entitled, "Reevaluating the Miracle Cocktail" he writes:

Protease inhibitors have not stopped my need for God's Love We Deliver. Nor my need for a part-time home aide. And certainly not ADAP. As all these professionals speak out on television and in print about new hope, going back to work, getting off benefits, what class of people do we as long-time survivors surviving in spite our damned debilitating symptoms become? Failures? Unclean? Tough-luckers? Poor? (1997)

Morris' account reflects the views of people with HIV/AIDS who have not been "cured" by medications and their concerns that being ill will mean they are forgotten or turned away. On a broader level, Patrick Califia-Rice critiques the emphasis that has been placed on finding a cure in the fight against HIV/AIDS. He recalls the experience of seeing people's health fail on protease inhibitors, despite the promise of a cure that is often associated with new drug advancements:

it was horrible to see friends feel better for a few months only to slide back into pain and panic. Nevertheless, many of us bit like wide-mouthed basses in 1996 when David Ho, MD, predicted that protease cocktails would perform the same miracle. (2001)

The concept of eradication — "a fancy word for cure" — emerged from and contributed to the "End of AIDS" ideology that was prevalent in the late 1990s. In order to counter this myth and provide accurate information about treatment options, personal testimonials and overviews of clinical research were used in PWA publications to show that HIV could not be eradicated through the use of protease inhibitors and combination therapy.

A second medical scientific advancement in the mid 1990s contributing to the "End of AIDS" ideology was the introduction of viral load testing. Simply put, a viral load test measures the amount of HIV in a person's blood (a low measure ranged from 400-500 copies depending on the test and a high measure could be in the hundred of thousands). The term "undetectable" was used to describe when the level of HIV in a person's blood was below the threshold of the test. Like the term eradication, an undetectable viral load became associated with the elimination of the virus from the human body.

> In the Vancouver afterglow, two words — undetectable and eradication — took on totemic powers. The near-mystical allure of undetectable virus — and eradication fantasies — was so compelling that people at all stages of disease rushed to seek treatment … . Friends who had started on anti-HIV therapy for the first time were told by their doctor just weeks later that their virus was now "undetectable." "Does that mean I'm cured?" they demanded. (Barr, 1997)

In this article by Mike Barr he describes the experiences of a person with HIV/AIDS who tries to use protease inhibitors — ritonavir — with the goal of improved health and an undetectable viral load.

> Geoff's viral load had fallen from the mid-200,000 range to 2,000. … And outside the ritonavir moments [side effects], he noticed an increase in energy. In another two or three months, if he was lucky, the virus in his blood would vanish. Because viral-load tests can only measure HIV levels of 400 to 500 (copies of HIV RNA per milliliter of blood) and above, it has become common to refer to viral load below this arbitrary cutoff as "undetectable," the new holy grail of AIDS docs worldwide. Geoff hoped soon to refer to himself,

in the strange way that others with such levels now do, as "undetectable." (1997)

The viral load test was adopted by health care professionals and people with HIV/AIDS as a primary marker of their progress in managing their illness. Medical technologies like viral load that are used to measure disease progression, while a useful clinical tool, have influenced the self definition of people living with chronic illness (Flowers, 2001). Viral load measures, especially if the result was undetectable, became for many people with HIV/AIDS a new way of understanding themselves in relation to the virus and a sign of their success or failure. As one person with HIV/AIDS wrote, "in 1996 my viral load never went above 20,000 so it's been a good year" (Martin, 1997).

In the late 1990s, activists, treatment advocates and people with HIV/AIDS began to write about how undetectable viral load measures could misleadingly give the impression that someone was cured or rid of the virus. In her attempt to dispel myths about protease inhibitors, Karin Timour wrote in *Body Positive*,

Myth #3: If your viral load is undetectable, you can't transmit HIV, so you don't have to worry about condoms. An undetectable viral load just means that the amount of HIV activity in your blood is less than our current tests can measure. Undetectable does not mean that one is HIV negative, nor does it mean one couldn't infect someone. (1997)

The concern was that people would misinterpret "undetectable" as meaning that they no longer had HIV and as a result were no longer infectious. This perception was further exacerbated when in April of 1997 Magic Johnson's wife Cookie announced to *Ebony Magazine* that her husband had been healed because his viral load was undetectable (Randolph, 1997). In apprehension about resurgence in the infection rate, prevention efforts in the late 1990s tried to dispel the myth that having an undetectable viral load result was a sign that you were cured.

AIDS Isn't Over: In December of 1998 *POZ Magazine* started to include on its cover the byline "Because AIDS isn't Over." This explicit countering of the "End of AIDS" ideology that had dominated discourses about the epidemic since the mid 1990s reflects a gradual shift, in accounts of living with HIV/AIDS, in the degree of optimism and hope regarding the potential of medical science to cure or eliminate HIV/AIDS. Mike Barr, who wrote extensively for several publications about HIV treatment options, wrote in early in 1997 that "we're in the honeymoon period with these drugs, and whether this is going to be an enduring marriage is unclear." Over the course of the late 1990s it became evident to activists and people with HIV/AIDS that protease inhibitors and combination therapy could not deliver on the promise that they held when first introduced. Using worries about the Y2K bug, David Salyer in late 1999 expresses the pessimism that followed the optimism from earlier in the decade:

> The other big millennium bug, HIV, will continue to defy eradication for the time being, creeping into the next century, invading bodies all over the world, wreaking havoc on lives. No matter what you may have heard, AIDS isn't over. (Salyer, 2000)

The new medications transformed people's lives, often for the better, but they turned out not to be a cure and they created new kinds of social and medical problems for people with HIV/AIDS. During the late 1990s a key theme in accounts of living with HIV/AIDS was to point out the consequences of making the assumption that we were in the twilight of the epidemic or that AIDS was over. Joe Greenwood makes this point in his lament about feeling burnt-out as person with HIV/AIDS trying to counteract the "End of AIDS" ideology in AIDS work:

> Many of us involved in the HIV/AIDS community are programmed to preach the gospel according to HIV: "Practice safer sex," "AIDS affects everyone," "We have not found the cure for AIDS," and of course, "AIDS isn't over!" While it is necessary to get these messages out to the public, sometimes the overwhelming amount of

things yet to be done, people yet to reached and the urgency of it all can leave you extremely burned out. (2000)

As with Greenwood's feeling of fatigue, there is a gradual shift in the level of optimism and hope in accounts of living with HIV/AIDS with regard to the potential of medical science to provide a cure. Instead, one of the main messages in the late 1990s was that HIV/AIDS continues to be a social and medical problem that requires an ongoing community based and institutional response.

Living with HAART

After 1996, with the advancement of protease inhibitors and combination therapy — what would become referred to as HAART, highly active antiretroviral therapy — living with HIV/AIDS became closely intertwined with using (or not using) medications. In this social climate, people with HIV/AIDS were expected, as much as was possible, to seek the expertise of health care professionals and take advantage of the quickly expanding treatment options available to them. Medical discourses that informed research and clinical care relied heavily on the restorative and transformative potential of HAART (Wong & Ussher, 2008). An underlying assumption behind emerging models of care was that HAART could and should bring patients back from serious illness (Persson, 2004) and enable them to survive with HIV/AIDS as a chronic manageable illness (Holtgrave, 2005). Writing for the Seattle Treatment Education Project, Andrew Elliot comments on the interrelationship that emerged in late 1990s between HIV and HAART:

The way that treatment is provided changes the way that people experience chronic illness. In 1997, more effective antiretroviral therapies now called highly active antiretroviral therapy (HAART) became the standard of care for HIV affected individuals. This therapy has changed the face of HIV, becoming part of the *language* of HIV infection, its care and treatment. (2003)

Accounts of living with HAART during the late 1990s in publications by and for people with HIV/AIDS reflected, to large extent, this imperative that those infected need to rely on institutional medical care and prescribed medications in the management of their illness — it is shown to be, as Elliot suggests, the language of living with HIV/AIDS. Yet, this imperative is not taken up uncritically. Writers and contributors to PWA publications sought to expand on this biomedical approach to treatment by drawing on their own experiences and perspectives of people using HAART. This critique of medicalization — which in this instance refers to the assumption that treatments and medical care alone was enough to survive — was expressed in relation to recurring themes about living with HAART: negotiating adherence/compliance and the risk of resistance to treatments; managing side effects and treatment holidays; and illustrating the work of people with HIV/AIDS who are trying to make informed treatment decisions often under difficult circumstances. Activists, educators and people with HIV/AIDS tried to illuminate the difficulties and challenges of using HAART in an attempt to offset the extent to which medical discourses surrounding the epidemic prioritized this treatment protocol.

Adherence and Resistance: One of the key challenges of HAART was that the medications needed to be taken as prescribed to be effective. Noncompliance meant that people with HIV/AIDS not only were not benefiting from the drugs, they were also at greater risk for developing resistance to the medications. Understandably, given the emphasis placed on HAART as the standard of care, adherence became a central issue for researchers, clinicians, AIDS service organizations and people with HIV/AIDS. Reflecting back at the XII International AIDS Conference in 1998 Mike Barr notes that,

> Geneva did pay attention to some of the emerging problems associated with treatment — particularly adherence. Treatment adherence was becoming a hot issue. Not only because it was causing large numbers of people to develop drug resistance, but also because the development of adherence services was a money maker for health care providers and community organizations — many of

whom were looking for new things to do since so many of their clients no longer required the kinds of late-stage AIDS services they were accustomed to providing. Adherence was the new "program." Not that there is anything wrong with that, but it was a little odd to see so many community-based organizations jumping on the treatment education bandwagon with such a vengeance after being reluctant for so many years. (2003)

Publications that were produced by AIDS service organizations, PWA coalitions and treatment advocacy initiatives, like Barr suggests, began to place more emphasis on giving people with HIV/AIDS the resources they needed to adhere to treatment regimes in order to make the most of HAART. Treatment information organizations, like Project Inform, warned that non-adherence could lead to increasing instances of treatment failure:

Reports about the successes of new treatments for HIV/AIDS have provided a welcome respite from the despair of recent years, but most recent data has begun to show increasing evidence that more and more people are beginning to fail on these therapies. ... How long treatments will last is closely connected to how well people adhere to the complex regimens required by the new drugs. AIDS service organizations must help people living with HIV understand the importance of adherence in maintaining the hope offered by the new drugs, and must help them develop methods to cope with the demands made by these drugs. (Staff, 1997)

Personal accounts by people with HIV/AIDS provided a slightly different perspective on the problem of adherence. Many protested that the regimes set out by pharmaceutical corporations and health care professions were extremely hard, if not impossible, to follow. Dispelling myths about protease inhibitors, Karin Timour, relating the experiences of John Hatchett, argues that in fact no one can follow the schedule set out by some treatment regimes:

Myth #4: No one follows those Crixivan food and drug schedules. It's not humanly possible. "You can't eat for two hours before you take it, or for an hour afterwards ... I take my first dose when I get up, and an hour later eat breakfast. Lunch is 1-2 p.m., so that at 4 p.m. I can take my afternoon meds (medications)." "I fear developing resistance, but I could make myself nuts. If something comes up to interfere with my scheduled meds, I give myself an hour's grace period. My goal is to get back on schedule as soon as possible. Say I wake up late, and take the first dose at 9 a.m., an hour later than usual. Using the grace period, I'd take my afternoon dose at 4:30 p.m., rather than 4:00 p.m., eat dinner from 5-10 p.m. and have my midnight dose on schedule. It's weird to feel incredibly normal, while keeping my food schedule in front of my mind." (1997)

The dietary and scheduling demands of HAART, especially the initial medication combinations and regimes, were such that people with HIV/AIDS often had to re-organize their daily lives around taking HAART. People with HIV/AIDS, like Luciana McCabe writing for the publication *Women Alive*, articulated the difficulties of using HAART.

The last thing I see every night before I close my eyes to go to sleep is a bottle of Crixivan. I swallow a couple of pills and try to ignore the burning sensation creeping up through my chest as I lay my head down on the pillow. ... The next morning the alarm wakes me up at eight and the first thing I see is the bottle of Crixivan. I swallow two more pills with the half glass of water leftover from last night and I get up. I know at 4 pm my wrist alarm will go off, screaming for two more pills, yet, I look forward to living one more day. (1997)

Yet, despite the difficulties in following regimes, many people with HIV/AIDS writing about their experiences draw attention to the importance of being compliant or adherent because the benefits outweigh the risks. McCabe goes on to write,

Monotonous and sometimes painful, the truth is that the triple drug combination I take is improving my health. Two years ago it was going down hill with no brakes. I now have more energy, more T-cells and more weight. I have a new job and have regained some control over my own life. (Instead of letting HIV control it). I feel healthier and happier. But, even though I am compliant, I know that other things may still go wrong. The threat of intolerance and resistance is still lurking around me and every other person on triple-combo. (1997)

As the "language of HIV" it would have been difficult for people with HIV/AIDS in the late 1990s to reject the idea of adherence as a key component of using HAART. The risks of resistance and intolerance were perceived to be too great. Instead, accounts of living with HIV/AIDS demonstrated just how difficult it was to be adherent and the social and life consequences of trying to follow very complex and demanding treatment regimes.

In depicting the work involved in following treatment regimes, people with HIV/AIDS in the late 1990s interrogated the distinction between compliance and adherence that was prominent during this period. The term compliance refers to the extent to which a patient is able to follow, more or less unquestioningly, the treatment protocol prescribed by their physician. Adherence, in contrast, refers to the extent to which patients follows a treatment regime that they have negotiated in partnership with their physician. Looking back at 1998, staff writers at *POZ Magazine* point out that many people with HIV/AIDS rejected compliance in favour of adherence.

Adherence. Sure, it sounds dull, but back in 1998 adherence was serious business. Historically, taking (or not taking) your meds has always been called compliance. However, in the grand tradition of PWA empowerment dating from those hallowed Denver Principles, AIDS activists, journalists and HIVers blanched at the term's "do what you're told" connotation. So our take-no-shit crowd insisted on the more active adherence. See also: the medically correct "You failed on your combo," which became "My combo failed me." (Staff, 2004)

Taking up the more active notion of adherence and rejecting the more passive compliance, even though it is not in opposition to dominant medical discourses, is consistent with the ethics of self empowerment.

From its origins in Denver in 1983, the PWA movement has centered around self empowerment for all people with HIV/AIDS. A key component of self empowerment is not to blindly trust one's health and well being solely to any physician, even one who is well respected and trusted; but rather to have a healthy degree of distrust that becomes translated into each patient, educating him or her self about the illness and treatment options, and once educated, deciding which treatments will be tried, *in partnership with the doctor.* (Shernoff, 1997)

HAART posed many challenges for people with HIV/AIDS in the late 1990s. The new treatments were promoted as a chance to recover from illness and to live longer with HIV/AIDS. At the same time, HAART was very hard to take and missing doses or not following schedules could mean becoming resistant or intolerant to existing or future medications. Adherence during this period was described and understood as a strategy, ideally, which enabled people with HIV/AIDS to actively participate in treatment decisions along with their physician even though using the treatments was often very disruptive and complicated. Unlike compliance, the burden of responsibility for adherence was not carried solely by the patient. Portraying the difficultly of using the treatments sent the message that medical science and the health professions could fail patients by expecting them to engage in treatment regimes that were unreasonably difficult. Making the challenges of adherence visible and known made way for the new treatments and treatment regimes that were more consistent with the lives of people with HIV/AIDS.

Side Effects and Holidays: Not long after the optimism following the Vancouver conference in 1996, an increasing number of stories began to emerge from people with HIV/AIDS using the medications detailing the experience of often severe and debilitating side effects. Initially accounts of sickness caused by HAART were seen to be a minor setback in relation to the dramatic effects of the drugs on many people's health. Over time, though, it became apparent that side effects were becoming a serious health burden for people using HAART.

After living in the shadow of death for over a decade, the AIDS community heralded the protease era with frenzied exuberance. Awakening from this interminable nightmare, those at the brink arose from their deathbeds to contemplate a future once again. Amid the celebration, the specter of long-term side effects was overlooked, as any side effect seemed preferable to death. But unbeknownst to us, a monster lay sleeping, about to rear its ugly head. The honeymoon with HAART (highly active antiretroviral therapy) was tarnished as reports of bizarre side effects began accumulating. (Grinberg, 1999)

By the end of the 1990s the number of accumulated side effects possible from the use of HAART was remarkable. Lark Lands in *POZ Magazine* (2000) identified the following *categories* of side effects that could result from HAART: appetite loss; body distortions; bone death; diarrhea, fatigue, gas and bloating, hair loss, insulin resistance and diabetes, kidney stones, muscle aches and pains, nausea, neuropathy, night and daymares, pancreatitis, skin sins (rashes). The purpose of Lands' article was to help people with HIV/AIDS understand and manage the different types of side effects that result from the medications.

One of the institutional side effects of the medicalization that occurred post-HAART, was reluctance among professional authorities to recognize the emerging difficulties with the new medications. PWA publications in the late 1990s became one of the only forums for people with HIV/AIDS to express their experience of side effects. As Linda Grinberg notes in her article "Honeymoon to HAARTarche" accounts of side effects became central to the language of living with HIV just as advancements in new medications had become the new language of HIV in the late 1990s.

Complaints of protease inhibitor-associated diarrhea, gas, nausea and heartburn — euphemistically referred to as "ritonavir moments," ... — were soon matched by stories of people on indinavir (Crixivan) winding up in the ER, waiting in agony for "kidney sludge" to pass. ... But the phenomenon that came to overshadow all others, causing PWAs the most angst, is a host of inexplicable changes in body shape. ... New catchwords entered the HIV lexicon: crix belly, visceral fat, buffalo hump, truncal obesity and protease paunch. Yet none of these terms fully capture the human misery. (1999)

Profiles in PWA publications in the late 1990s also detailed the experience of side effects. People with HIV/AIDS profiled were often asked to comment on their approach to using HAART. The response often included a reference to blood work test results like viral load and side effects. An example is an article on Canadian activist Louise Binder. When asked "are you taking any drugs" she responds:

> I've been on Crixivan, d4T and 3TC for about three years now, and the combination seems to be working. I haven't been sick at all. My blood work numbers are good, and I have an undetectable viral load. (Minnich, 1999, p. 87)

Like Binder, achieving an undetectable viral load was portrayed by many people as the defining marker of success when using HAART. This success, however, was often accompanied by stories of sickness and disfigurement from side effects. Binder continues her account:

> But I have had a lot of side effects with these drugs. Some of them come and go, like hair loss. ... I have a buffalo hump from the Crixivan, which goes away and comes back. The lipodystrophy has made my legs extremely thin, while my breasts have enlarged incredibly, and I have no waist to speak of. Also my face has gotten very puffy along the jaw line, which looks odd ... . I also have gastrointestinal difficulties, which nothing seems to help, some peripheral neuropathy and elevated triglycerides, which I'm told is also a side effect from the drug combination. (Minnich, 1999, p. 87)

It was common for people with HIV/AIDS, in their accounts of using medications, to celebrate institutionalized medical markers of improved health, such as viral load test results. Yet, medical advancements often required compromising quality of life. While in most portrayals of side effects they were presented as manageable, soon many people with HIV/AIDS began to seriously question whether they are willing to sacrifice their well being for increases in immune function and the amount of virus in their bodies.

At this point in the epidemic, advocates and activists with HIV/AIDS had began to regularly contribute to magazines like *Body Positive*, *POZ Magazine*, and *Positively Aware*. Jim Pickett, who regularly writes for *Positively Aware*, described his experiences of using HAART:

> The HIV didn't make me sick until I started on the meds that are going to help keep me well. Now this is the one that really gets me. Oh super. I felt great, but there it was in black and white, the disease was progressing, numbers don't lie, better do something about it. So I finally succumbed, to the mantra of "hit hard, hit early," to the strange glamour of cutting edge HIV therapy, to those ubiquitous ads that made me think I'd be hot and buff and glossy, shooting the rapids in a kayak, if I only were cocktailing. So I signed up. What choice did I have? (1999)

The notion of eradicating HIV from the human body fuelled an approach to HAART that Pickett describes as "hit hard and hit early." Only after further research on the medications did scientists and clinicians realize that this approach would not work and causes people severe side effects. This scenario is what happened to Pickett, as he describes:

> But my sun dappled technicolor fantasies on how I would triumph over this wily virus were usurped by the opposite of "glossy," which I guess might as well be called reality. ... The only "shooting rapids" I've dealt with have been diarrhea.... Exciting, unpredictable diarrhea. Farts gone terribly wrong, split-second timing marking the difference between "fresh" and "soiled." If glamour is nausea, fatigue and headaches, gagging, choking, farting, and burping, then call me CoCo cuz I got it down cold, dahling. Puke is the new puce. High collars are back, the better to camouflage that lipodystrophy that's become so popular. Ah shucks, sarge, I may be able to climb to the mountain top and shake my fists at the sky, but I'm gonna have to rip down my cargos and frantically squirt a nuclear, membraneous gruel from betwixt my firm glutes as

soon as I get there. But hey, I've got well over 700 CD4s and the
virus remains undetectable. (1999)

The tension described by Pickett between staying with HAART and
suffering the consequences or giving up the medications and running the
risk of serious illness brought on by the disease was the impossible
scenario that many people with HIV/AIDS had to face when making
treatment decisions. It led many to consider taking a drug holiday, a term
that quickly became integral to the HIV lexicon. Another writer with
HIV/AIDS, Joe Greenwood, wrote an account of his first "drug holidays":

At the end of last year, the "cocktail" of antivirals that I was on
started producing some rather severe side effects. I found out first
hand about lipodystrophy when my belly got huge, making me
actually look pregnant. More frightening, though, were the strange
things that began happening to my kidneys — my blood test results
went haywire, and my doctor actually had to send me to a renal
specialist. When I suddenly passed a bladder stone for the first time
in my life, my doc and I decided it was time for me to come off the
cocktail for a while, and look into a different combination I could
try. I went on my first "drug holiday." (1999)

Greenwood finds that once he stops HAART his side effects diminish and
he starts feeling better without drastic drops in his blood test results, as he
feared. Also, Greenwood notices that many of his HIV positive friends
were also on drug holidays.

I found out that a lot of other people I knew were on drug holiday
as well, something I hadn't paid a lot of attention to before. Most of
them were off the antivirals for the same reason I was: they had
simply run out of drug combos, and were waiting for new drugs to
be approved. But while I was speaking with them, I noticed that,
like me, they seemed to be looking and feeling better than they had
in a long time. Most of them were worried about their viral loads
going up, too, but they all commented on how nice it was to be free
of the side effects. (1999)

Based on accounts by people with HIV/AIDS the incidence of a physician sanctioned drug holiday, as was the case with Greenwood, was unusual. Many people with HIV/AIDS stopped their medications for a brief period or reduced the dose on their own accord to alleviate side effects or to lengthen the time before they became resistant to available combinations of medications.

What is also unusual about Greenwood's account is his endorsement of taking voluntary drug holidays occasionally in order to find relief from side effects. By and large, the message from accounts in PWA publications was that side effects, though horrible, were manageable and better than facing opportunistic infections from a compromised immune system. David Morris' account is more typical in warning against the dangers of drug holidays.

> My AIDS drugs make me sick, but I take them anyway. It would be great to take a "drug holiday," but I don't dare because I don't want my viral loads to skyrocket and I don't want my virus to become resistant to my medications. Sometimes I get tired of taking my medications, which are little daily reminders that I have a disease for which there is no cure. I miss not being able to drink my morning coffee until I've eaten my breakfast and taken my pills. I miss the freedom of being able to come and go as I please without worrying when and where I'll take my medications. But HIV doesn't take a holiday, so neither do I. It's difficult, but it's worth it, because I've seen what can happen when HIV-positive people don't take their medications. (2001)

The issue of whether it is legitimate to take a holiday signaled an important broader struggle around standards of care regarding the use of HAART. People with HIV/AIDS voicing their concerns about the debilitating side effects from the medications served as a call for professional authorities to reconsider the "hit hard, hit early" approach combination therapy and the unquestioning adoption of HAART. As the decade came to a close, there was more debate about alternative strategies for using HAART that could be just as effective without compromising people's health. One approach, for instance, that came about from observing the experiences of people with HIV/AIDS, became referred to as "Structured Treatment Interruption, or STI, the first snappy AIDS acronym of the new millennium": essentially taking drug holidays under the supervision of your physician in order maximize the benefits and minimize the hazards of HAART (Delaney,1999).

Treatment Sophistication = Survival: A central tenet of the PWA self empowerment movement is being involved in the decisions that affect your life. This involvement is especially poignant when it comes to health and health care decisions. Collectively, people with HIV/AIDS involved in the PWA movement have cultivated a collective lay expertise drawn from their experience of living with this disease. As Epstein (1991) has shown, this knowledge was influential in reforming policies regarding clinical trials and drug research development in the 1990s. Research on approaches to treatment and care has shown that people with HIV/AIDS cultivate their own expertise, and rely on the expertise of peers, when managing their illness (Adam & Sears, 1996). One ongoing objective, perhaps even the primary objective, of PWA publications has been to cultivate and share the knowledge of people living with HIV/AIDS.

In the late 1990s the development of HAART intensified the need for people with HIV/AIDS to acquire an extensive knowledge of the medical management of HIV/AIDS. People with HIV/AIDS had to learn a new and very complex language of treatment and health care options often with little guidance from health care professionals who themselves were also encountering a very steep learning curve of quickly evolving standards of care. Accounts of living with HIV/AIDS during this period chronicled the experience of having to make complicated treatment decisions regarding adherence and side effects often under very difficult circumstances.

I take twenty pills a day. Sixteen of which are enormously enormous. Glaxo gets all thrilled with itself when it combines AZT and 3TC into one pill, Combivir. I say big deal, those pills were tiny to begin with. ...Why do sixteen of mine, those protease inhibitors called Agenerase, have to be big enough to gag even the most talented of throats? Why the hell can't they combivir those suckers? ... Twenty pills a day, that for the first several months made me sick to the gills, and still do to this very moment as I write this, just not as severely. Twenty pills a day that are helping contribute to the very real threat of deforestation I pose via my generous, ongoing use of mass quantities of toilet paper. Twenty pills a day that remind me how "sick" I am, keeping me tethered, enslaved to the idea of "disease." Ah the emotional and mental battles. Can I do this forever? Can I take 7,300 pills a year, endlessly? Can I remember every time? Can I resist the temptation to skip, to indulge in a drug holiday here and there? Can my body tolerate it all? And what will happen when it can't? (Pickett, 1999)

Accounts of managing treatment decisions, like this one, often stressed the complexity and uncertainty of using HAART. The way that many people tried to deal with this situation was to become more actively involved in their health and health care. Having to adapt to the quickly changing landscape of managing HIV is what Sean Strub refers to as treatment sophistication:

Larry Kramer estimated in the March issue of *POZ* that there are 5985 different possible anti-HIV drug combinations now available; data are being collected on only a few. ... Even with the data we do have, it is alarming that so many doctors inappropriately prescribe combination therapy. Some experts have called for a special licensing requirement for physicians to prescribe anti-HIV drugs; others have suggested an intensive education requirement for patients to receive the therapy. A tiny cusp of us who are unlucky enough to have HIV but lucky enough to have money, education and time to become treatment sophisticates now have a shot at survival. TREATMENT SOPHISTICATION = SURVIVAL. (1997)

In the late 1990s publications like *POZ* concentrated on providing treatment information and advice in an attempt to give people with HIV/AIDS the tools to educate themselves about HAART. At this time the PWA organizations began to make use of the Internet as a forum for disseminating information about treatment and health care options. One of the key issues that emerged at this time was the sequencing of drugs;

helping people with HIV/AIDS to understand what drugs to take and in what order so as to maximize the long-term benefits of HAART.

> To hear some drug companies, doctors, researchers and publications tell it, deciding on the best strategy for choosing among the 15 approved anti-HIV drugs and their thousands of possible combinations is simply a matter of good science and clear thinking. In reality, picking an effective, long-lasting combo is more like playing the one-armed bandits in Las Vegas. And, on top of choosing a first-time combo, HIVers must face the added complexity that each choice made upfront affects the options available later on if the combo fails. This issue has recently been dubbed "sequencing" — mapping out which drug combo to use first, which to switch to for No. 2 and which to save for No. 3, 4 or more. (Delaney, 2001)

An ongoing concern in the advice given by and for people with HIV/AIDS was that professional authorities — public officials, drug company executives, physicians — could not be fully trusted to act in their best interests. In the case of physicians, for instance, it was simply that many, unless they specialized in HIV, were unable to keep up to date on the latest practice guidelines regarding HIV treatment and care.

> The proliferation of new medical options for people with HIV comes as a welcome respite. ... Yet the very expansion of options has made treatment decision making more difficult. For many, the sense of urgency about treatment decision making and timing creates a potent anxiety. Complicating this is the reality that while standard therapies have been published, many physicians, especially those who are not HIV specialists, are unsure about or unfamiliar with them and fail to adequately manage patients with HIV. As a result, people living with HIV/AIDS are faced with the need to make a number of decisions about treatment: whether or not to begin combination therapy; when to do so; whether to change treatments in response to an increase in viral load or intolerable side effects; and, in some cases, whether to stop combination therapy. (Shernoff & Smith, 2000)

In response, profiles of people with HIV/AIDS stressed the importance of being involved in health and health care decisions. The message was that it is necessary to take the guidance of health care professionals but ultimately you needed to be in control of treatment and care decisions.

> "Before, I didn't really care to know anything about HIV. I let my doctor do the work, and I just did what he told me." Now Mark takes part in the decisions that affect his health, retaining the ultimate yea-or-nay over his treatment regimen. "I think it's important to take responsibility for yourself," he says. "My friends and my family definitely played the most important role in my recovery, but a close third was me taking active part in my care." Knowledge is power, and sometimes it is life itself. (Staff, 1999)

Personal accounts by people with HIV/AIDS expressed the often frustrating and at times empowering experience of being more reliant on medicine and medical care yet having to question the expertise of their physician.

> You can no longer be totally dependent on doctors and drugs to engage this invader. This experience fortified me and gave me a new resolve. I re-learned what a formidable force of nature we are capable of being. So, use the resources at hand. Rest. Build yourself up. Never abdicate responsibility and watchfulness again. (Courson, 1999)

One of the key factors that created feelings of distrust of professional expertise was the extent to which institutional authorities had an investment in HAART, if not as a cure, then as an effective means to treat HIV/AIDS. Stories about the difficulties of adherence, the torment of side effects, and the work of managing illness pointed out that protease inhibitors, combination therapy and HAART had flaws that were not being acknowledged quickly enough in the institutional response to the epidemic. Furthermore, the necessity for people with HIV/AIDS to become "treatment sophisticates" in order to survive created a situation of disadvantage for those who had fewer resources — like education, social class, occupation, or social support — to draw upon when trying to become more actively involved in their health care decisions.

The AIDS Industry

Prior to the development of HAART, the business of HIV/AIDS consisted primarily of companies — sometimes referred to as viaticals — that bought the life insurance policies of people with HIV/AIDS who thought they would not live very long. Selling life insurance came back to haunt some of those infected as they realized that HIV/AIDS was not the death sentence that was portrayed in early representations of the disease. In the 1990s, as health promotion for people with HIV/AIDS became more prominent, progressive health and nutrition based businesses like NAYA began to advertise with publications like *POZ*. At this time the fashion industry also began to take up HIV/AIDS as a way of raising their profile, selling clothes, and demonstrating that they were socially responsible. Still, for most of the epidemic, mainstream businesses have avoided HIV/AIDS because of the stigma of the disease. Sean Strub, the founder of *POZ*, commented in the *New Yorker* magazine that his publication would be a success the day a car company like Ford or General Motor bought advertising:

A lot of advertisers don't want to associate their brand name with a disease ... . One day, *POZ* will probably run an ad for a car company. What a statement of support ... (Lubow, 1995)

The term "AIDS industry" usually refers to the institutional collaboration between medicine, government and drug companies that emerged in the 1990s as more effective medications were developed and HIV/AIDS became a profitable disease. Even though the AIDS industry relies on a triad of social institutions it is the drug companies, justifiably, that have been targeted by treatment activists and people with HIV/AIDS as taking advantage of and profiting from the epidemic. Since the beginning of the epidemic, those involved in the PWA movement have articulated a distrust of social institutions that extended to include businesses and industries. However, a specific critique of the AIDS industry was formed in the 1990s when it came to be known that early medications, AZT most notably, were ineffective in treating HIV but did cause serious, and potentially irreversible, side effects.

The distrust of drug companies and the AIDS industry generated in the early 1990s carried over when protease inhibitors were announced at the International AIDS Conference in Vancouver. Before the conference began, members of ACT UP New York had already articulated a strategy around the slogan "GREED=Death ~ Access for All," a play on the familiar early slogan "Silence=Death," which targeted drug companies who were seen to be limiting access or profiting unreasonably. At the opening ceremony of the conference Eric Sawyer said to participants

> Yes the preliminary results from these hugely expensive combination treatments look great. But we are a long way from a cure, even for the rich who can afford the treatments. ... To the drug companies, people with AIDS say it's time to drop your prices. Drug companies should consider developing a two tier pricing system that allows reasonable profits to be made from the rich. But, AIDS treatments must also be made available to the poor everywhere, at cost or at very minimal levels of profit. And if you drug companies don't make this shift voluntarily we will advocate for governmental regulations to mandate this and fight to have your patents taken away from you. ... GREED = Death, end the greed. Demand Access to All. (1996)

With the initial success of combination therapy and HAART the critique that was so strongly present at the conference dissipated but did not disappear. Soon after the conference, activists and people with HIV/AIDS began to write about their concerns regarding the effectiveness of the new medications and the hype that was being generated about them. In article entitled "The Morning After" Mike Barr warned about overemphasizing the benefits of HAART:

> The protease inhibitors have unquestionably infused with new life many people desperately in need of powerful anti-HIV treatment. In the absence of a cure, though, the finite benefits of these new drugs should be employed strategically — with the aim of conserving as

many therapeutic options as possible, as first choices fail and lead
to second choices, and second choices fail and lead to third. (1997)

As the decade unfolded, and the realities of adherence, resistance, side
effects, and intolerance became more evident, this critique of the AIDS
industry gained momentum. In PWA publications during the late 1990s
concerns about the AIDS industry took several forms. Activists and people
with HIV/AIDS wrote about drug companies misrepresenting the benefits
of HAART without due consideration to the dangers and risks. As people
with HIV/AIDS began to question the benefits of HAART more emphasis
was placed on the viability of alternatives like complementary medicine
in the management of HIV/AIDS. Lastly, the excess profiteering from the
use of HAART was raised as a major impediment to people with
HIV/AIDS receiving medications.

Marketing HIV/AIDS: After 1996, once it was evident that protease
inhibitors and combination therapy held promise as a treatment for HIV
— at least for many people — drug companies began to aggressively
market the new medications. In what would come to be a controversial
advertising campaign, the drug company Merck promoted its drug
Crixivan with images of healthful young men and women hiking on the
summit of a mountain. In an article on the marketing of HIV drugs,
Richard Goldstein interviewed the designer of the advertisement about its
evolution and design:

Like many successful ad campaigns, this one evolved over time
from adversity to triumph. It began in 1996 with a climber staring
at the rock face before him. ... Subsequent ads showed the same
climber helped to the summit by a hunky black man. And then he's
on top, standing with a proud black woman against a pure blue sky.
(Never mind the shifting cast of characters — this is an equal-
opportunity fantasy.) "They don't have their hands in the air," says
Buford. "We didn't want to communicate that science has found a
cure." Instead, the copy reads, "If you're HIV+ Crixivan may help
you live a longer, healthier life." A plausible message, but it pales
before the deeper meaning of the quest. You're clawing to stay

alive, the imagery suggests, but with this drug you can stand at the summit, looking down. (1998)

Activists and people with HIV/AIDS critiqued this advertisement, and AIDS drug campaigns like it, because it misrepresented the benefits and underrepresented the potential dangers. One person with HIV was quoted as saying, "I'm doing pretty well on your drugs but when am I going to look like a mountain climber" (Hattoy, 1998). The AIDS industry, it was argued, was selling a fantasy — the promise of a longer healthier life — without sufficiently warning about the potential pitfalls. In the same article Goldstein goes on to argue that

> To some extent, this is a plausible promise. (If it weren't, the Food and Drug Administration, or FDA, which regulates direct-to-consumer drug advertising, could prevent such claims from being made.) But it's hardly the whole story. Though the ads mention side effects, they give little sense of how deep the downside of these drugs can be. Only when you read the fine print ... will you discover that the "contraindications" may be severe, even fatal. "I know a lot of people taking these drugs who have experienced the Lazarus effect," says veteran ACT UP/New Yorker Eric Sawyer. "But I also know a lot of people who have had their hair fall out, and their skin color go from light brown to a really horrendous gray." (1998)

Pharmaceutical companies countered this criticism by pointing out that they regularly use HIV positive individuals in their advertisements. Advertisements for the medication Viramune, for instance, feature a photograph of the HIV positive crew of the racing yacht *Survivor*. Yet critics like Goldstein argue that the point isn't as much about realism as it is not creating a portrait of treatments that might led people with HIV/AIDS to make decisions that could be detrimental to their health, by using medications when they would be better to wait. On the prevention side, questions were also raised about the extent to which drug advertisements contributed to a culture in which people no longer felt that HIV posed a serious health risk.

Responding to the fantasies portrayed in drug campaigns came in part through the personal accounts of side effects from people using medications like Crixivan. Even though many PWA publications featured such advertisements, and benefited financially from them, they continued to publish stories about the difficulties of using HAART. Not long after protease inhibitors became widely used, for instance, the drug Crixivan came to be known in portrayals by people with HIV/AIDS as a drug that was potentially effective but painfully difficult to take and often came with severe side effects. One article by Ken Miller was entitled "Starving to Death to Live: Crixivan — The Newest "Silver Bullet" in AIDS Treatment!" (1996). Another account by Pat Rolands told of kidney damage from using the drug.

> I am writing this article because of my recent hospitalization resulting from the popular protease inhibitor, Crixivan. The "side-effect" I suffered from this drug was complete blockage of my left kidney, almost causing kidney failure. ... Since my hospitalization, I have heard that kidney sludge is being seen in other people who are taking Crixivan. They are being told that the way to prevent this is to drink more water. ... People on Crixivan are also being told to be certain that their doctors are doing regular urinalysis. (1997)

Rolands believes that her side effect came about, in part, because drug companies do not sufficiently take in consideration the differences between men in women in clinical trials. Historically women have not participated equally in clinical trials and this has led to their health needs being neglected. According to Rolands,

> we know that there are not enough women in the clinical trials. Not in any clinical trials. But there are some. And the drug companies have the data. We need and we have the right to have that data analyzed by gender. Our lives depend on it. (1997)

In addition to clinical trials, people with HIV/AIDS raised concerns about the reliability of information provided by the drug companies regarding the risks associated with their medications. Stephan Gendin takes exception with feeling as if the AIDS industry is not being honest with those whose health is at risk from using HAART:

> Besides the side effects themselves, the thing I hate most about taking my pills is the drug company propaganda that the side effects aren't so awful and fade away over time. Having spent years on AZT monotherapy with no complaints, I know that is sometimes true. But since going on the triple combination therapy in 1993, the side effects seem to grow with each passing day. So, it royally pisses me off when I encounter what feels like a massive conspiracy to minimize the consequences of swallowing large quantities of often toxic medicine. I would rather be dealt with honestly. (2000)

Similarly, Dave Gilden wrote about the dangers of people with HIV/AIDS and AIDS activists tacitly embracing the AIDS industry as the means by which to manage the disease. In the late 1990s, clinical trials of the drug Lodenosine were halted after the death of participants (Rodriguez, 1999/2000). Gilden advocates for a more skeptical approach to dealing with medications and drug companies:

> With current anti-HIV meds taxing bodies to the limit, activists have pressured pharmaceuticals to churn out better treatments. The lodenosine scandal should give us pause. Above all, it is a wake up call to HIVers not to trust companies to provide complete, objective information about dangers. Drugs need careful evaluation, not reckless promotion. Nobody sounded the warning bells over lodenosine — not even activists or independent researchers. We must never take anything for granted again. (2000)

Gilden identifies the point of view expressed at this time that many activists and people with HIV/AIDS were complicit in looking to the AIDS industry to provide the answer to the treatment of HIV/AIDS. In the late 1990s, accompanying the critique of the "End of AIDS" ideology and the pursuit of a medical scientific cure was an acknowledgement by those in the AIDS movement that they had a role to play in this process of medicalization, of pushing unquestioningly for a medical solution to a complicated social problem.

Complementary Medicine: When people with HIV/AIDS began to seriously question the promise of HAART many started to consider the role of complementary medicine in promoting health and managing illness. The use of complementary medicine is not a new trend in the treatment of HIV/AIDS. In the late 1980s and early 1990s alternative and complementary therapies were quite commonly used by people with HIV/AIDS (Pawluch, et al, 2000). There was a resurgence of interest in complementary medicine in the late 1990s as distrust in scientific medicine increased and people started to look for health care alternatives to HAART. Reports from a conference on integrative medicine began:

> Two decades into the AIDS pandemic, we finally seem to be starting to agree that there is more to treating HIV than searching for a magic pill, or an enchanted drug cocktail. AIDS has proven to be the health problem of our age — the disease that challenges western biomedical science's toxic approach to healing. (Sacks, 1999)

As in the case of integrative medicine, which combined a range of different approaches to health, complementary medicine was not portrayed in PWA publications as an alternative to HAART. In the special issue of *POZ* on alternatives, the editors began: "We're not saying, 'hop off the protease express and jump on the bitter-melon bandwagon.' We just don't want you to settle" (Editor, 2000). Not wanting to settle aptly expresses the view of complementary medicine as an approach to health that gives people with HIV/AIDS options that they would not otherwise have by only relying on scientific allopathic medicine. In some cases, not settling meant combining together "western and eastern" modalities in treating HIV/AIDS, as in this profile:

> [Laura] began to have vision difficulties, and balance problems kept her from walking well. Nonstop diarrhea combined with inability to eat resulted in serious weight loss. She was bed-bound for several months. Her family aggressively sought answers, and finally, NIH researchers diagnosed inflammation in the brain caused by HIV. Lara was placed on potent antiviral drugs (acyclovir and foscarnet) for almost a year. Her family believes that it was the

combination of these with complementary therapies—especially nutrients—that ultimately brought her back. Today, Lara still uses the best-of-East-and-West approach. She's a healthy teenager living her life the way she wants to. And she credits her survival to the circle of family around her. (Lands, 1998)

In other instances the use of complementary medicine was a more direct challenge to scientific medicine and HAART. In 2000, *POZ* profiled seven people with HIV/AIDS who have refused to use medications and instead have opted to use a range of alternative modalities. One woman, Chardelle Lassiter, remarks about her approach:

A voice deep inside me eleven years ago told me not to take antiretroviral drugs — that they were toxic and would not work for me. I have learned to respect that voice. I attribute my success to that spiritual strength. [My doctor and I] have the same conversation at every appointment. She says "go on the drugs," and I say, "No, I'm not ready." It's our little ritual. (Staff, 2000)

The views of Lassiter and the six other people with HIV/AIDS profiled reflect a reaction against the "hit hard and hit early" approach to the use of HAART that was prominent after protease inhibitors were introduced. Taking this attitude often required actively challenging the advice of professional authorities and the message from the AIDS industry about the advantages of HAART. It also required challenging the conventional view of complementary medicine as acceptable so long as it is used as an additive rather than equivalent treatment modality. Or, in other words, alternative health care is acceptable provided that it is used to alleviate side effects or help with adherence to a treatment regime. As editors of POZ who introduced the profiles wrote, many people with HIV/AIDS were no longer seeing complementary medicine as just an "add-on":

What if, as our profilees profess, alternative treatments are not just "harmless add-ons" to HAART that make you feel a bit better but powerful tools for PWA survival? And while we're tweaking conventional wisdom, let's leave no theory unturned. What if HIV is only one of many cofactors causing an immune-system crisis?

With the eradication boom gone bust and researchers refocusing on immune rebooting, these questions are as cogent as ever. (Staff, 2000)

In accounts by people with HIV/AIDS complementary medicine was seen to offer a greater range of health care options that were perceived to be beneficial on many levels: less toxic and not driven by profit; health promoting and not illness producing; and involving being active and taking more control of decision making.

The turn to complementary medicine opened up less toxic modalities for people with HIV/AIDS than HAART. At the same time, health care alternatives also gave legitimacy to the illness experiences of people with HIV/AIDS. In an article on the myths associated with the dominance of scientific medicine in the late 1990s, Sean Strub argued for recognizing a range of different types of evidence about what works in managing HIV:

> Myth #7: Anecdotal evidence doesn't matter. It does. Especially to people with HIV, who put more faith in what they hear from other people with HIV than in what they are told by AIDS organizations, government agencies, drug companies or health care providers. When the science establishment starts responding to people with HIV by conducting the studies we want — on drug, herb and supplement combinations and a whole host of complementary therapies — the faith may move back to the scientific literature. But until then, we'll rely on each other. (1996)

Strub is writing when the excitement about HAART was at its height in the mid 1990s. With the emphasis placed on adherence and viral load in maximizing the medical benefits of HAART, the experience of illness became secondary to markers of disease progression. The affinity between complementary medicine and illness experiences helped to legitimate an approach to managing HIV that was based on feelings as well as blood tests.

> I'm not just basing the stabilization of my health on new drugs — there's no way I'd do that. We supplement these heavy medications with a lot of alternative treatments: We're now taking echinacea,

vitamin C, cat's claw [a Latin American herb], grape seed extracts and a multiple that includes vitamins A and E and bee pollen. I take these complementary therapies to balance out my body. I'm not looking for any specific effect — I just want to restore my body to normal after putting all these toxic drugs in it. I have walking pneumonia right now, and the herpes is still spreading. Physically I'm a little fatigued. But emotionally I feel fine! And to tell you the truth, I don't give a fuck about my labs. If things feel good, things are good. (Martin, 1997)

The approach of this woman to managing HIV/AIDS is a combination of HAART and a range of complementary therapies. It reflects the conventional view that medical scientific treatments are toxic yet necessary and that complementary medicine can balance the side effects of medications — help her to become normal. Yet, this perspective privileges, or at least places equal value upon, the experience of illness in relation to clinical measure of health. As the pursuit of eradication lost its legitimacy, and people with HIV/AIDS began to realize and experience the negative aspects of HAART, complementary medicine was perceived as a challenge to the preoccupation of those involved in the AIDS industry who privileged and relied on an approach to managing HIV that was organized around the use of HAART and the legitimacy of scientific medicine.

Greed=Death: Returning to the slogan by ACT UP from the International AIDS Conference in Vancouver, a third critique of the AIDS industry by activists and people with HIV/AIDS was that medications were overpriced. The greed of drug companies was leading to needless suffering and death. One version of this critique stated that the cost of medications limit access and drain resources from already overburdened social and health care services.

Welcome to the brave new world of pharmaceutical roulette, where a dicey mix of exorbitant prices, inadequate insurance and dwindling public-health services keep powerful, potentially life-extending drugs out of reach for thousands who need them. While

magazine headlines herald the supposed twilight of the AIDS
epidemic, many PWAs are left frustrated and angry because the
drugs they've been waiting and praying for — though on pharmacy
shelves — may not be available to them. (Lederer & Brownworth,
1997)

In this article, Bob Lederer and Victoria Brownworth raise concerns about
the injustice when people with HIV/AIDS are unable to affordably access
medications: "While destitute PWAs get sick — and die — for lack of
treatment access, investors thrive on pharmaceutical stocks." They point
to the need for activists to continue calling for transparency, pressuring
pharmaceutical industries to declare the amount that they profit from the
AIDS medications.

While some people with HIV/AIDS perceived the medications as life
saving and lack of access as the corruption, others felt that AIDS
industries were also unnecessarily and dangerously promoting the "End of
AIDS" ideology of eradication through HAART:

I have felt like shit for the last two and a half years.... Why am I
making my life so exceedingly difficult, ball-and-chained to
decidedly non-recreational drugs when I am basically healthy? Why
am I not saving these drugs for when they will do me the most good,
when the risk of nasty side effects is actually less than the benefits
I will obtain? Why am I on state aid to receive these drugs? (I
couldn't possibly pay for them after my clinical trial ended.)
Because doctors and large, multinational pharmaceutical companies
still actually push the agenda of "eradication" via the obsessive need
to keep the viral load "undetectable." Why is that? ... Well, there is
a lot of money to be made. My simple little regimen of 18 pills per
day runs about $12,000 a year — some pretty good coin. (Pickett,
2000)

The difficulties of using HAART combined with overly optimistic
marketing campaigns created a situation in which people with HIV/AIDS
began to seriously question the motives of drug companies. In accounts of
living with medications pharmaceutical corporations came under scrutiny

for profiting from medications that, while potentially beneficial, also created serious health problems for people with HIV/AIDS.

The success of HAART and the resulting medicalization heighten the position of pharmaceutical industries as key players in the institutional response to the epidemic. Eradication lent legitimacy to the idea that pharmaceutical industries had the capacity to create an effective long term treatment for HIV/AIDS. The institutional "fight against HIV/AIDS" became more about funding medical solutions than it was about addressing broader social, political and cultural dimensions of the epidemic.

> The high price of drugs is destroying what there is of the dismal U.S. public healthcare system. AIDS Drug Assistance Programs (ADAP) have been crippled nationwide and the formularies of state Medicaid programs are under enormous strain. The pharmaceutical industry protests that they run a risky business and that their prices are fair. There's nothing wrong with drug makers earning a fair and decent profit, nor, certainly, with researchers bringing home good pay for doing good work. But with government subsidies, tax write-offs and the numerous incentives industry receives in the form of corporate welfare, the profit from bringing a drug to market dramatically outweighs the cost. (Carter, 2002)

A version of this situation in the United States can be extended to Canada and indeed most western industrial democracies. Yet, as the decade ended, many activists and people with HIV/AIDS felt disillusioned with the extent to which the AIDS industry would put the needs of those living with HIV/AIDS over profit and corporate self interest.

> I'm still clueless here in 1997. In 1986 I had great hope for AIDS to be the divine equalizer. Unfortunately I remain disillusioned. AIDS has divided where it should have united. It has invoked greed where compassion is far more appropriate; it has given new energy to the old vendettas of the perpetually self-centered. It has given birth to a new breed of opportunists capitalizing on the suffering and vulnerability of the dead and dying. It has given new meaning to incompetence in the workplace known as the AIDS industry. It has given countless exploitive capitalists permission to steal AIDS

funding when pure greed or a personal agenda is their objective
motivated by race, sexual, or substance user's causes. It has
manifested the ugliest in human nature, even though it was an
invitation to all of us to go to a higher place. Most of us haven't.
But we still can. (Horowitz, 1997)

This account by Robin Horowitz was entitled "1987: Silence=Death;
1997: Apathy=Death." It reflects a growing concern among activists and
people with HIV/AIDS in the late 1990s that self empowerment and
community development had diminished with the rise of the AIDS
industry and HAART.

The HIV community must unite in demanding an end to the price
spiral for existing drugs and an end to increased price thresholds for
new drugs. There is perhaps no more critical domestic battle around
HIV than the fight to stabilize, if not reduce prices. Without it, our
entire system of paying for medical care for people with HIV is in
jeopardy, brought about by the companies that already profit most
from the disease. (Delaney, 2002)

A central component of the AIDS industry critique articulated by activists
and people with HIV/AIDS was to reverse the trend toward
commercialism. This call for a renewed community response was not a
rejection of HAART and the AIDS industry. Rather, it was an effort to
influence the discourses that created meaning about the real benefits of
HAART and the social consequences of investing in medical treatments
as a means of responding to the epidemic.

Conclusion

In the introduction to *Surviving and Thriving with AIDS*, an early guide to
living with the disease, Michael Callen remarks that "whenever people
with HIV/AIDS get together, talk always turns to treatments. And when
we are done talking about treatments, we talk about treatments some
more" (1987, p. 45). In the mid 1990s, the development of protease
inhibitors and combination therapy promised to deliver what treatment
activists and people with HIV/AIDS had been advocating for since the

beginning of the epidemic: an effective and safe medical treatment. Up until this time medications like AZT were available but caused difficult side effects and were found to be of marginal benefit for most people with HIV/AIDS. It appeared as if — as was announced at the International AIDS Conference in Vancouver — the new medications were able to drastically improve the health of people with HIV/AIDS and increase their chances at long term survival. The protease era represented a time of hope and optimism that was amplified in institutional discourses to the level of anticipating the "End of AIDS" and the eradication of the virus.

In this chapter I have chronicled the response — the talk about treatments — of those involved in the PWA movement to the medicalization of HIV/AIDS that resulted from the ascendancy of medical science as the accepted institutional means to address the epidemic. There were three main themes that predominated. One was an engagement with the "End of AIDS" ideology that emerged in institutional discourses in anticipation of medical science developing a cure for HIV. Activists and people with HIV/AIDS initially embraced the success of the new treatments, celebrating the miraculous recoveries of individuals who returned to health after taking the medications. At the same time, accounts of living with HIV/AIDS also highlighted the difficulties that accompany a renewal of health for people who had anticipated not surviving for a long period of time. Another element of the "End of AIDS" ideology that people with HIV/AIDS both embraced and questioned was the idea of eradication. Viral load testing emerged at this time and was used by those infected and by health care professionals as markers of disease progression. Medical markers assisted in measuring the replication of HIV yet it also tended to diminish the illness experiences of people with HIV/AIDS and misconstrue the capacity of medications to eliminate HIV entirely from the body. While many accounts by people with HIV/AIDS praised the benefits of the new treatments, it soon became evident that it was necessary to counter the "End of AIDS" ideology by demonstrating that the medications were not as effective as initially thought and that those infected were still becoming ill and dying.

A key element of this critique was to highlight the difficulties that people with HIV/AIDS experienced using HAART. Accounts of living with HAART were concerned with the extent to which professional authorities prioritized adherence as a necessary component of taking medications without much consideration to the — at times — impossibility of following treatment protocols. In addition to adherence, people with HIV/AIDS also experienced considerable side effects and eventually began to question the long term viability of using HAART. The complexity of HAART and the preoccupation of professional authorities on the benefits of the new medications, or their inability to keep up with current research, created a situation in which people with HIV/AIDS had to acquire their own knowledge and expertise regarding managing illness. Fortunately, PWA and AIDS organizations responded by providing vast amounts of treatment information through publications and the internet. However, taking advantage of this resource required a certain level of social and cultural capital — education, money, social support — that was not available to all people with HIV/AIDS.

The last theme that was predominant in the late 1990s was an expanding critique of the AIDS industry. Activists and people with HIV/AIDS have always governed a skepticism regarding medical science, the state, and drug companies. Despite the benefits of HAART for many people with HIV/AIDS, this skepticism continued, though many argued with not enough fervor, when drug companies began to use marketing strategies that misrepresented or over exaggerated the promise of the drugs without sufficient attention to side effects and health risks. As the decade unfolded and it became evident that HAART had severe limitations and that drug companies were generating large profits from the medications, activists and people with HIV/AIDS began to explore alternative treatment modalities like complementary medicine. Drug companies were also accused of overpricing medications and limiting access to those who could benefit from the medications. Despite this critique, there were many in the PWA movement and AIDS movement who believed that the commercialism of the late 1990s had generated complacency among activists and professional authorities; they claimed that too much attention was being devoted to drug development and scientific medicine and not enough on addressing the underlying social, political and economic factors that contribute to the epidemic.

In 1999 David Drake wrote a short article in *POZ Magazine* on the media entitled "When Plagues Return" (p.20). The main point that Drake makes is that the mainstream media, after celebrating the medical advancements in the mid 1990s and fueling the "End of AIDS" ideology, was just beginning to recognize "the new AIDS crisis" resulting from the shortcomings of HAART. In accounts of living with HIV/AIDS in the late 1990s it is possible to see two broad trends that are significant for understanding the PWA movement at this time. One trend is the extent to which writing in PWA publications followed the medicalization of HIV and concentrated on HAART and the experiences of people who were living the new treatment revolution. Medical science did become the language of HIV not only for professional authorities but for many of those living with the disease. Yet, the second noteworthy trend is that the engagement with medications was not done so uncritically. Activists and people with HIV/AIDS were able to draw on their own experiences in order to critique the negative aspects of HAART, articulate reforms to institutional practices, and find alternative ways of managing their illness. In this regard it is evident that the PWA movement helped to offset the ways in which medicalization misrepresented the lives of those using HAART and living with HIV/AIDS. The stories and accounts of people with HIV/AIDS demonstrated how the "End of AIDS" ideologies and the move toward scientific medicine and commercialism were not the sole means, or even the best means, by which to address the epidemic.

Chapter Four

GLOBALIZATION, 2000-2006

This chapter examines a period of globalization in the HIV/AIDS epidemic that began in the late 1990s. The possibility of HIV/AIDS becoming a global pandemic was recognized not long after the first cases were identified in the United States and in equatorial Africa in the early 1980s (Iliffe, 2007). By mid decade, cases were reported in most regions of the world and it was evident that the epidemic would be difficult to control (Knight, 2008). Government officials, scientists and health professionals from numerous nations (albeit most were developed, industrialized democracies) met in 1985 at the first International AIDS Conference in Atlanta, Georgia to discuss the scope of the epidemic and what might be done in the way of a response. In 1988, the World Health Organization initiated "World AIDS Day," recognized each year on December 1st to raise awareness of the epidemic as a global problem (World AIDS Campaign, 2008). By the beginning of the 1990s the *New York Times* predicted, based on epidemiological studies, that "by 2000, there will be 10 million cases of AIDS worldwide, 90 percent of them in developing countries, principally among the impoverished"(Altman, L. K., 1991, p 4). Despite this knowledge, governments and international organizations like the World Health Organization and United Nations were slow to respond sufficiently on a global level given the magnitude of the pandemic (Knight, 2008).

In North America the PWA movement initially began in large metropolitan cities like New York, Vancouver, Toronto and San Francisco. Despite this local orientation, organizers and activists built national and international networks based on the tenet that HIV/AIDS is a crisis that cuts across geographic and socio-political boundaries. Soon after the declaration of the Denver Principles in 1983, the National Association of People with AIDS — which had ties with organizations in Canada — was initiated. In the late 1980s, international coalitions like the Global Network of People with HIV/AIDS were formed to address the rapid worldwide spread of the disease and advocate for a wider global institutional response to the pandemic. In 1995, the seventh international conference for people with HIV/AIDS was held in Cape Town, South Africa and concentrated on human rights and community development in endemic countries. International PWA initiatives like the Global Network were influential in raising awareness about the need for a more concerted global response to HIV/AIDS in endemic countries. Over the 1990s, as rates of infection in developing nations continued to climb exponentially while rates in developed nations leveled out, national and international authorities came under increased pressure from organizations like the Global Network to formulate a more concerted response to the global AIDS epidemic. In 1996 the Joint United Nations Programme on HIV/AIDS (UNAIDS) was initiated to improve the global institutional response to the epidemic. By the late 1990s, it became widely acknowledged by institutional authorities that HIV/AIDS needed to be defined as a crisis that was global in proportion and perpetrated by the inequities and injustices that exist between developed and developing nation states.

In this chapter I chronicle the portrayal of HIV/AIDS as crisis of globalization in publications by people with HIV/AIDS. I begin with the 13th International AIDS Conference (2000) in Durban, South Africa,which was a pivotal moment in shifting toward the treatment of HIV/AIDS as a global pandemic. This is followed by a discussion of initiatives within the global PWA movement. Organizing during this period of the epidemic began to coalesce across geographic and socioeconomic boundaries. Building on this discussion, I trace a number of issues — treatment neglect, women with HIV/AIDS and AIDS denialism — that emerged as a result of the globalization of the epidemic. The chapter concludes with an analysis of how the shift in orientation toward a global pandemic has transformed the PWA self empowerment movement.

13ᵗʰ International AIDS Conference: Global Manifesto

During the late 1990s, as rates of infection continued to escalate in developing countries, especially Africa, there was an expanding urgency about the adequacy of current responses to the global epidemic. This viewpoint reached a crescendo at the 13ᵗʰ International AIDS Conference in Durban, South Africa. Described as the "conference of century" the meetings in Durban have come to be seen as a global wake up call to the severity of the pandemic and the need to address HIV/AIDS as not just a medical issue but one that is linked to inequalities across nation states. One person with HIV/AIDS who attended the conference wrote in *POZ Magazine*:

> "Bridging the Gap" was the official theme of the 12th World AIDS Conference in 1998, but that meeting merely gestured toward the chasm between the globe's treatment haves and have-nots. At No. 13 in Durban in July, the first such affair ever held in a developing country, the gap swallowed the conference whole. With Africans constituting a third of the 12,437 delegates (by far, the largest proportion ever), there was no escaping a painful irony: High-tech studies on viral resistance and future meds were irrelevant to many of the doctors and PWAs in attendance. ... There's no doubt that No. 13 was the scientific conference gone political, a reminder that AIDS has always been as much about society as about science. (Wright, et al., 2000, p 1)

From the perspective of participants (officials, health care professionals, activists, and people with HIV/AIDS), hosting the conference in Durban, and seeing how the epidemic was unfolding in Africa first hand, led them to realize the extent to which HIV/AIDS had become a global crisis. Another account of the conference noted that:

> The 13th International Conference on AIDS, held in Durban, South Africa, proved to be both the most important and the most unusual meeting since the earliest days of AIDS. This is the first time that the huge international meeting has been held in the heart of the

global epidemic. More than any previous conference, one was forced, by pure proximity, to confront the most rapidly escalating human suffering associated with the disease. It riveted attention on the prohibitively high cost of drugs and the need to build the medical and social infrastructure required to support the complex treatment of HIV. Similarly, it provided an important watershed for many African countries, a time to fully acknowledge the threat they face, to ponder the cost of government inaction and the need for clear thinking about solutions. (Project Inform, 2000, p. 1)

One of the key messages from Durban was that the benefits from treatment advances that people had enjoyed (with the caveat that HAART or highly active antiviral therapy was not always beneficial) in North America and in other developed nations were not accessible to the multitude of people with HIV/AIDS in poorer countries where the epidemic was growing. In 2000, the problem extended beyond simply making medications more accessible; the social and political infrastructure of poorer countries needed to be improved so people had the means by which to take advantage of advances in the treatment of HIV/AIDS.

This year's XIIIth International AIDS Conference in Durban, South Africa was not the typical AIDS conference. Because of the pressing social needs faced by developing nations, the emphasis of the meeting was not primarily directed toward biomedical research and studies. Instead, the main topics of discussion included human rights, reducing the stigma faced by people living with HIV, prevention, vaccine research, access to care, reduced drug pricing and building medical and social infrastructure. (Project Inform, 2000, p. 1)

Discussion of stigma, development and human rights regarding the global response to HIV/AIDS were taken up the media and contributed to raising awareness among the public in developing nations about the severity of HIV/AIDS in poorer countries around the world. After the conference, the editor of *Body Positive* Raymond Smith wrote a series of articles reflecting on the pandemic. A year after the conference Smith argues that the Durban conference did help to create a more global conception of HIV/AIDS in developed nations.

He began the series by commenting that

> Ever since the International AIDS Conference in Durban, South
> Africa, in July 2000, world attention has been riveted on the rapid
> expansion of the HIV/AIDS epidemic across the globe. Of course,
> troubling news had been coming out of Africa and other regions of
> the world for some time. But the hosting of the conference in Africa
> highlighted the growing disparities between the developed world,
> where antiretroviral therapies are increasingly available, and the
> Third World where they remain largely unknown. (Smith, 2001, p.
> 1)

The Durban conference gives us a glimpse into the social context of
HIV/AIDS at the end of the 1990s. Accounts of the conference serve as a
barometer of the institutional response to HIV/AIDS and the state of the
PWA movement at this moment in the epidemic.

One major reason for hosting the 13th International AIDS Conference
in Durban, South Africa was that institutional authorities in developed and
developing nations had begun to recognize in the late 1990s that not
enough had been done to address the spread of HIV/AIDS in poor and
endemic countries. According to Poku (2002), the Global Programme on
HIV/AIDS (GPA) formed through the World Health Organization in 1986
— the central organization in charge of formulating a multilateral response
to the global epidemic — had been ineffective on several fronts. One
criticism was that initiatives under the GPA did not sufficiently take into
consideration the underlying social and political factors contributing to the
increase rate of infection in endemic countries. Further to this, Poku
(2002) notes that another limitation was

> a growing dissatisfaction among donor governments with the
> working of GPA, seen as hamstrung by its place within WHO and
> unable to work effectively with other UN agencies. This was further
> complicated by the structural weakness of the WHO: particularly in
> developing effective strategies, coordinating policies and providing
> financial support for activities at the country level that would slow
> down the transmission rates of the virus. (p. 116)

In an attempt to redress the deficiencies in the GPA, the joint United Nations Programme on HIV/AIDS (UNAIDS) was formed in 1996. Building on the work of its predecessor, UNAIDS set in place what turned out to be a more effective series of strategies designed to improve the international response to treatment, advocacy and education. Poku (2002) has identified four areas in which the UNAIDS has been successful: (1) they put in place systems for gathering and acting on surveillance data on the spread of infection in specific countries that took into consideration socioeconomic and political factors; (2) they relied more on programs that target behavioral factors like unprotected sex or injection drug use without clean needles that put people at greater risk of infection; (3) they advocated to have HIV/AIDS a greater priority within the political agenda of participating countries; and (4) they lobbied for the inclusion of direct stakeholders into the governance of specific initiatives in countries and in the programme in general. Leading up to Durban, UNAIDS helped to set the foundation for understanding HIV/AIDS as a global crisis that has been severely neglected and deserves serious attention among institutional authorities in developing and developed nations.

> Several years ago, the idea of holding the 13th International Conference on AIDS in South Africa seemed like a great idea. It made perfect sense to move the conference to one of the great epicenters of the epidemic. The focus on South Africa, and Durban in particular, became fairly obvious. It was not only the right country but also the right city, one of few in the developing world that had the capacity for managing such an event. Moreover, as the wealthiest country facing AIDS in sub-Saharan Africa, there was reason to hope that bringing the conference to South Africa would be preceded by serious prevention and treatment programs that might then serve as examples to the rest of Africa and Asia. (Project Inform, 2000, p. 3)

The Durban conference, as suggested in this account by the treatment organization Project Inform, was one effort — important because of its profile and the worldwide attention it is given, primarily through its coverage in the international media — in a series designed to further draw attention to the global AIDS crisis in areas of the world in which it is endemic and hopefully spark further efforts to improve prevention and treatment efforts.

Increased awareness generated by a renewed international response put the governance practices of endemic countries under a level of scrutiny that was not in place earlier in the epidemic. Just prior to the Durban conference, this issue was amplified when the president of South Africa, Thabo Mbeki, began to make claims questioning whether HIV was the cause of AIDS. In one report on the conference, it is suggested that Mbeki's reliance on the claims of HIV dissidents and denialists was based primarily on his naivety, indicating the lack of dialogue between public officials and scientific and medical experts across developing and developed countries:

> The outlook for the conference was confounded when South African President Thabo Mbeki stumbled into the camp of the AIDS denialists while out cruising the Internet. President Mbeki's intrigue with denialist theories caused many scientists in Africa and throughout the world to wring their hands in despair and even cancel plans to attend the meeting. Though it is clear that Mbeki made a big mistake in giving a platform to the denialists on a pre-conference panel he created, it is equally clear that he raised some critically important questions that must be addressed if Africa is ever going to be able to cope with AIDS. Unfortunately, too much attention has been focused on his involvement with discredited fringe theories. Lost in the debate are the true challenges he has raised about how to bring solutions to his country. (Project Inform, 2000, p. 4)

The comments made by Mbeki, and the credibility that he afforded to individuals and groups who question the relationship between HIV and AIDS, generated a strong and widespread reaction among conference participants. During the conference a group made up primarily of health care professionals and scientists drafted the Durban Declaration, a document refuting claims that HIV does not lead to AIDS. The declaration begins by setting the global context of HIV in 2000:

Seventeen years after the discovery of the human immunodeficiency virus (HIV), thousands of people from around the world are gathered in Durban, South Africa to attend the XIII International AIDS Conference. At the turn of the millennium, an estimated 34 million people worldwide are living with HIV or AIDS, 24 million of them in sub-Saharan Africa. Last year alone, 2.6 million people died of AIDS, the highest rate since the start of the epidemic. If current trends continue, Southern and South-East Asia, South America and regions of the former Soviet Union will also bear a heavy burden in the next two decades. (Smith, 2000, Declaration section, p. 1)

Much of the document cites research that reaffirms the link between HIV and AIDS and outlines the importance of concentrating on HIV as the best means to direct treatment and prevention efforts. At the end of document, the delegates reassert the claim that science will eventually provide the means to curtail the spread of HIV/AIDS.

There is no end in sight to the AIDS pandemic. By working together, we have the power to reverse the tide of this epidemic. Science will one day triumph over AIDS, just as it did over smallpox. Curbing the spread of HIV will be the first step. Until then, reason, solidarity, political will and courage must be our partners. (Smith, 2000)

The document was signed by "5,018 physicians and scientists from 82 countries who are dedicated to the control of HIV/AIDS" and garnered worldwide attention to the global AIDS crisis and problems that may exist in the political governance in endemic countries (Smith, 2000). This declaration became one of the key markers of the conference and began, arguably, a renewed sense of solidarity and political commitment among scientists and health care professionals — a group that has been criticized since the beginning of the epidemic for their apolitical stance with regard to the epidemic — across developing and developed nations.

The shifting tide toward understanding HIV/AIDS as a global crisis began to extend to the medical industrial complex in the late 1990s. Advancements in the treatment of HIV/AIDS with the development of protease inhibitors in 1996 had transformed the economics of the disease because pharmaceuticals corporations were able to develop, market, and profit from HIV/AIDS medications. Coinciding with the success in the business of treating HIV/AIDS was the exponential spread of the disease in poorer countries around the world. Leading up to the conference in Durban, governments and pharmaceutical corporations came under increasing pressure to develop strategies to ensure that treatments for HIV/AIDS could be made available to people living with HIV/AIDS in endemic countries. In an account from the conference by a group of people with HIV/AIDS noted that

> the conference's mantra was first sounded at the opening plenary, when South African judge Edwin Cameron, an openly positive HAART-taker, made a ferociously moving call for universal access to antiretrovirals. Debates on treatment access dotted the program, while even at clinical-science sessions the audience raised the issue again and again. With several demonstrations against drug-price gouging — also the hot topic of hallway conversations — pharmaceuticals were on the defensive. The usual Broadway-budget display booths were scaled-back productions this year, many "tastefully" papered with photos of African children. Almost every day, one company or another trumpeted drug giveaways for poor countries — often with strings attached. (Pfizer's free-fluconazole offer, for example, was limited to people with meningitis in South Africa and for only two years. (Wright, et al., 2000, p. 1)

While policies and regulations to make treatments more available and affordable had been promised and initiated one of the key messages that came from the Durban conference was that the drug companies and governments were not doing enough. There was frustration over the failure of prior efforts, like the following from 1998:

> A United-Nations sponsored pilot program to make powerful new AIDS drugs available at subsidized prices in Ivory Coast, first greeted with optimism, has quickly caused frustration among patients and medical officials. The majority of the 1 million HIV-positive people in the Ivory Coast will be excluded because

participants still face prohibitive costs for the drugs — $15,000 a year for each patient in a country where the per capita income is only about $500 — with the course of treatment lasting a lifetime. (Bornhoeft, 1998, p. 9)

A viewpoint that was articulated clearly at Durban was that the medical industrial complex needed to be held to ethical business regarding providing access to treatments to people in countries who cannot afford them. This pressure was coming increasingly from not only activists but all stakeholders in the pandemic as, for instance, countries like Brazil began to challenge patent legislation and started producing their own generic versions of AIDS treatments. (James, 2000)

Events at the Durban conference indicated that governments, international agencies, health care services, scientific research and even drug companies were beginning to adopt a more global orientation toward the HIV/AIDS pandemic. This trend was welcomed though treated with a measure of skepticism and cynicism among those involved the PWA movement and AIDS activism. Gregg Gonsalves, an activist and person with HIV/AIDS commented on this issue, drawing on his experience at the conference:

I think the whole meeting was a challenge to people, to researchers and activists alike, to actually look in the face at an epidemic of a proportion they've never seen before — to see the reality of AIDS in the developing world. Different people are going to rise to the challenge in different ways — and not rise to it. The challenges are enormous. Before we went to Durban, nobody could have predicted that the issue of treatment access in the developing world would have blown up to be such the hot button political issue of the meeting. (Treatment Action Group, 2000, p. 18)

An awareness of the global implications of the HIV/AIDS epidemic has been a longstanding theme in the PWA movement and AIDS activism. Two of the demands made by ACT UP and AIDS ACTIONS NOW! at the International AIDS conference in Montreal in 1989 was the establishment of worldwide treatment and prevention initiatives:

(6) Criteria for the approval of drugs and treatments should be standardized on an international basis so as to facilitate worldwide access to new drug treatments. (7) International education programs outlining comprehensive sex information supportive of all sexual orientations in culturally sensitive ways and describing safer sex and needle practices and other means of preventing HIV transmission must be made available. (AIDS ACTION NOW! & ACT UP New York, 1989)

In the years prior to and following the Montreal conference, several important initiatives were developed to help facilitate community development among people with HIV/AIDS across nations. Altman (1999) has noted that, while falling short in some respects, the GPA established in 1986 has played an important role in helping to build infrastructures among affected communities based on the principles of empowerment and self-determination:

Building on the strengths of local and national community organizing around AIDS, GPA encouraged the formation of networks such as the Global Network of People Living with AIDS (GNP Plus), the International Council of AIDS Service Organizations (ICASO) and the International Community of Women Living with HIV/AIDS (ICW). (p. 566)

The formation of international and global networks of people with HIV/AIDS assisted in sustaining within the PWA movement an awareness that more attention needed to be devoted to addressing the pandemic on a transnational basis. While not a prominent theme in the 1990s, this global orientation is evident in PWA publications in the form of news and updates regarding the spread of infection and the lack of a concerted international response.

By the close of the 1990s, there was in place an emerging and expanding global network of people living with HIV/AIDS ready to mobilize around the conference in Durban, South Africa. It was made up of both activists and people with HIV/AIDS from developed and developing nations. At the 13th International AIDS Conference, the key focal point for people with HIV/AIDS and activists was the need for global access to affordable treatments and the social and political infrastructure necessary in order for infected communities to benefit from them. Treatment for All was the title of the manifesto read at the conference by ACT UP:

> We are united with a single purpose, to ensure that everyone with HIV and AIDS has access to fundamental rights of healthcare and access to life-sustaining medicines. AIDS has become a catastrophe that threatens the very future of this planet. Terribly high levels of HIV infection and death due to AIDS are now a reality (rather than merely a projection) in poor communities worldwide. More than half of all these infections occur among women. AIDS is causing widespread devastation in Africa and Asia especially. THIS WAS AVOIDABLE. It is the consequence of negligence, particularly on the part of "first world" governments whose resources could have been mobilized to come to the practical assistance of poor nations many years ago. Political authorities have preferred to neglect public health, taking for granted the exorbitant cost of treatment, refusing to implement measures necessary for the strengthening of health systems, and prohibiting countries from setting up local medication production or from importing treatments essential for the survival of their populations. (ACT UP New York, 2000, p. 1).

The march organized by South Africa's Treatment Action Campaign (TAC) prior to the conference was another important event that signified an expanding political mobilization among people living with HIV/AIDS. That the march was made up of and organized by people with HIV/AIDS and activists from poorer nations was a sign that the movement was not just limited to the United States and developed nations. An account of the march in TAGline began:

> In May 1998, Ms. Gugu Dlamini was stoned to death in Durban for revealing that she was HIV-positive. A few days ago, 5,000 people, many wearing "HIV Positive" T-shirts, gathered at the Durban City Hall to demand equitable access to HIV/AIDS treatment. The excited group of nuns, drag queens, sangomas, doctors, communists,

teenage punks on skate boards, Pan-Africanists, gay activists, unionists, students and nurses had come from all over Durban, South Africa, and the world to join the Global March for Access to HIV/AIDS Treatment. The official posters castigated the drug companies for making huge profits from the AIDS crisis while the homemade posters said things like, "AIDS is as real as cancer" and, "Mbeki, forget your R3 million jet and buy us medicine." (Treatment Action Group, 2000, p. 1).

There were concerns expressed among delegates living with HIV/AIDS and activists that too much attention was being placed on treatments at the expense of broader issues like the determinants of the health, community development and prevention. Despite such concerns, reports from the conference by people with HIV/AIDS shared the view that the Durban meetings had helped to generate a greater global awareness among those involved in the PWA movement and AIDS activism.

The Global AIDS Epidemic

In the late 1990s the terrain of HIV/AIDS began to shift as the chasm in the incidence of HIV infection across the developed and developing world became apparent. Compounding this awareness was the gap in the means to health for people with HIV/AIDS living in different parts of the world. Commenting on the globalization of HIV/AIDS, John S. James, in his publication *AIDS Treatment News*, wrote that,

World consciousness on the HIV epidemic in developing countries — about 90% of the global epidemic — has changed greatly in the last three years. In 1998 the World AIDS Conference in Geneva took the theme "Bridging the Gap" — meaning the gap between access to treatment in rich and poor countries. But outside the conference there was no institutional support for saving lives in poor countries; once the speeches were done, that was it. And we all knew it. (James, 2001, p.1)

Looking forward after the Geneva conference and the Durban conference, Raymond Smith, the editor of *Body Positive*, described the future of HIV/AIDS as a global crisis as being between hope and horror. By horror he refers to the societal costs of HIV/AIDS in developing nations and the lack of response by governments, corporations and international agencies. As a counterbalance to the horror, though, is the hope that understanding HIV/AIDS in a global context in the PWA movement will help to generate more effective multilateral treatment and prevention initiatives.

> Perhaps most importantly, the conference did in the end succeed in bringing the catastrophe of AIDS in Africa to the attention of the world. Many conference attendees, in fact, reported that they had witnessed a sense of urgency and a revitalization of activism not seen for most of the 1990s. A potential disaster had somehow muddled its way to success. (Smith, 2001, p. 26)

As the trend toward globalization takes root, organizing among people with HIV/AIDS responded by, as Smith does, drawing attention to the forms of hope and the continued horror with regards to the pandemic. In the following sections, I trace several prominent themes in PWA publications between 2000 and 2008 regarding the portrayal of organizing among people with HIV/AIDS and the global AIDS crisis. The first looks at the PWA movement in developing nations and the emerging global network of people with HIV/AIDS. In the second section I examine accounts of emergent issues arising from the globalization of HIV/AIDS: (1) treatment neglect and accountability in developing nations; (2) a growing awareness of the gendered nature of the pandemic; (3) and the controversy that was generated surrounding the Durban conference about the rise of AIDS dissidents and denialism and the implications of this trend for responding to the global AIDS crisis.

PWA Organizing Worldwide

The International AIDS Conference in Durban drew attention to emergent forms of organizing and activism among people with HIV/AIDS. On one level, this organizing and activism occurred among those from the developing world who had, after being to Africa or hearing about the situation there via the conference, came to a different understanding of the pandemic. In an overview of the research from New York scientists, Derek Link makes this point when he wrote:

> Few Americans who attended the Durban AIDS meeting left without a profound of sense of transformation. AIDS activists marched through the streets of Durban, and the country's newspapers and televisions were dominated by AIDS coverage. The American advocates who attended the meeting spoke of feeling energy similar to the beginning of AIDS activism here, but in a wholly different context and with a wholly different set of challenges. Many left with broadened notions of what is possible in the fight against the global AIDS pandemic. (Link, 2000, p. 1)

The transformation that Link mentions led to a more careful and in-depth portrayal of the epidemic as it was unfolding in developing nations. Rather than one pandemic it became common to refer to many epidemics, a recognition that the social context in which illness occurs is important. Accounts of the pandemic after 2000 and the Durban conference also began to pay more attention to emergent organizing among people with HIV/AIDS in endemic countries. This awe at organizing and activism in developing nations can be seen in David Barr report from the Durban conference:

> After the meeting, there was a large rally outside the City Hall, organized by TAC. Union leaders, church leaders, activists, and even Winnie Mandela addressed the crowd. Thousands of people were wearing T-shirts that had "HIV POSITIVE" in large letters on the front. This alone was a chilling piece of activism as we were only 30 miles from where a woman was stoned to death for publicly declaring her HIV status. After the rally, we marched through the streets of Durban, yelling for treatment access. People were singing songs and dancing in the streets in a scene that was so reminiscent of all the anti-apartheid demonstrations I had seen on television. It was thrilling to be surrounded by South Africans demanding access to treatment and demanding that their government and all the

governments of the world address the AIDS crisis in Africa and worldwide. The march was peaceful, but very exhilarating. (Barr, 2003, p. 5)

Just as self-determination and a commitment to health from below was essential to the PWA movement in North America in 1980s, the same ethic was seen to be central for organizing among people with HIV/AIDS in poorer countries around the world. A key component to this self empowerment was facilitating the continuation of the networks of people with HIV/AIDS that had been put into place in the 1990s with the assistance of international agencies.

Global Epidemics: One of the purposes of publishing by those in the PWA movement has been to educate affected communities, institutional stakeholders and the public about the epidemic. Since the late 1980s, this education included keeping track of the spread of HIV/AIDS around the world. In this respect PWA publications served as a "media watchdog" with regard to the spread of the disease. One key source of information was delegates attending international conferences. David Barr, for instance, reported back from a conference in 1994 that

> among predictions of the rise in AIDS orphans and reports of the continued ascent of heterosexual transmission in this country, we will learn how one in three heterosexual men (and almost inevitably their wives) in the northern regions of Thailand have become infected with an especially virulent HIV strain transmitted through their weekly unsheathed visits to Thai prostitutes. We'll learn, too, how in India male truck drivers are bringing HIV home to their wives and families at an alarming rate. (Barr, 1994, p. 4)

AIDS activists and people with HIV/AIDS in the 1990s warned through news and information updates about the spread of HIV and about the need to address the epidemic as worldwide crisis.

The meetings in Durban were significant in that they brought international attention to the epidemic in Africa. After this conference, institutional representations — especially the mainstream media — began to portray HIV/AIDS as being synonymous with Africa. Accounts of the international response to the global HIV crisis most often concentrated on the epidemic in the African continent. This attention to Africa as the focal point of the global AIDS crisis was evident in accounts by activists and people with HIV/AIDS, though arguably before Africa came to dominant mainstream media coverage of the epidemic. *POZ Magazine*, for instance, devoted an entire issue to the topic of AIDS in Africa just prior to the conference in Durban:

> As you read our "Inside Africa" issue, we hope you gain insights into what it's like to live with HIV without clean water or easy transportation, among war and starvation. We have tried to bear witness to the miracles that are happening as people come together with faith and determination to save their families and villages from the ravages of AIDS. Our hope is that this issue will challenge the sincerity of AIDS activism and our responsibility as members of the global community. And force us to ask the hard questions. What is this fight about? Is the goal of the "AIDS movement" to eliminate HIV worldwide or to further widen the gap between north and south, rich and poor, black and white? These questions should be on our minds as we approach the 13th World AIDS Conference in July 2000 in Durban, South Africa, the first to be held in a developing country. (Wilson, 1999, p. 11)

In contrast to mainstream media, writing about the epidemic in developing countries by activists and people with HIV/AIDS — this 'bearing witness' — sought to portray more of the complexities of the crisis. One component of this complexity was an attention to the social and political circumstances that set the broader context for HIV/AIDS in different African countries. A section of the special issue of *POZ Magazine* challenged the assumption that all countries in Africa were incapacitated by HIV/AIDS.

> All of Africa is not an AIDS catastrophe. From Senegal in the west to Uganda in the east to Zambia in the south, certain governments took early and effective action. Even in hardest-hit Zimbabwe, individuals have come together to make miracles. (Editors, 1999, p. 1)

This series of articles describes the response of social institutions and communities to HIV/AIDS in four different countries — Senegal, Uganda, Zambia, and Zimbabwe — in order to show a more diverse and optimistic portrayal of the epidemic in Africa.

This attention to the specific social context of HIV/AIDS was also applied to accounts of HIV/AIDS in developing and developed countries around world. Raymond Smith, in *Body Positive*, goes so far as to question the utility of the term "the global AIDS epidemic":

> While it is common to speak of the "global HIV/AIDS epidemic," that term obscures as much as it enlightens about HIV in the world today. Consider that all forms of weather are, ultimately, part of one big "global" system — but that doesn't mean that the weather in Buenos Aires, Kuala Lumpur, and the Aleutian Islands have very much in common. And so, it is more accurate to speak of multiple, separate, if overlapping, AIDS epidemics as being part of one worldwide parallel pandemic. (Smith, 2001, p. 12)

Drawing on Mann and Tarantola (1996), Smith divides the epidemic into ten distinctive regions based on the spread of the disease, the social and political context, and the response to the epidemic. Once distinguishing "the worldwide parallel pandemic" he highlights four areas that have tended to be overlooked with regards to the HIV/AIDS crisis: Latin America and the Caribbean; North Africa and the Middle East; Northeast and Southeast Asia; and Eastern Europe and the former Soviet Union. He concludes the section by explaining the importance of attending to differences within the pandemic:

> Of course, even this division of the global AIDS epidemic into ten regions only begins to point out the multiple challenges posed by HIV around the world. But these subdivisions can at least suggest that beyond the AIDS epidemic we see around us in the U.S., and the horrible African plague we are increasingly seeing on television, exist many other complex — and equally urgent — AIDS crises. (Smith, 2001, p. 20)

Like in Smith, the portrayal of the "global AIDS crisis" among activists and people with HIV/AIDS included not only stories and articles about Africa but also many of the regions directly affected by the epidemic like Asia, Latin America, Eastern Europe and Russia.

By looking across the parallel epidemics, accounts by activists and people with HIV/AIDS draw attention to factors tied to globalization that contribute to the spread of HIV/AIDS across different regions. In his article Smith argues that "mass tourism, work migration, and refugee displacements account for a good deal of the world's exchange of people — and of HIV" (Smith, 2001, p. 28). Beyond the more fluid movement of populations, additional factors in the spread of HIV/AIDS were identified across many developing regions — like poverty and the ongoing stigma and homophobia associated with the disease. HIV prevention efforts in the Caribbean, for instance, are held back because of the stigma associated with the disease:

> Laws criminalizing homosexuality are still on the books in most Caribbean nations (in Guyana "buggery" is punishable by life in prison), exacerbating the region's violent homophobia, rampant HIV stigma and growing HIV infection rate (at nearly 2%, it is second only to sub-Saharan Africa). Caribbean governments, however, have responded to the dire epidemic with notorious sluggishness. ... With hate crimes occurring across the Caribbean ... some activists contend that [AIDS prevention campaigns] can't curb HIV rates until the governments pass laws to protect positive people's civil rights and medical confidentiality—so that everyone, gay and straight, can feel safe getting tested, seeking treatment and talking openly about HIV. (Villarosa, et al., 2006, p. 2)

In the years following Durban, the African continent emerged as a focal point for the expanding global AIDS crisis. Predominant in accounts of the developing countries by people with HIV/AIDS and activists during this period of time was the promotion of an understanding of the crisis as a series of interconnected though distinct parallel epidemics. Conceptualizing the "global AIDS epidemic" in this way was intended to provide a more accurate portrayal of the situation in developing countries and efforts within those countries, and to counter the overgeneralizations and obscurities contained in the mainstream portrayal of AIDS in Africa.

Global PWA Empowerment: The state and direction of organizing among people with HIV/AIDS was another key theme in accounts of the global AIDS epidemic. Attention to the global epidemic made activists from developed nations aware of community mobilizing around the world. Accounts of the epidemic post-Durban highlighted the efforts of people with HIV/AIDS in developing countries who were coming together to address their needs and bring about social change. One organization identified as a "success story" of activism in developing nations is the Treatment Action Campaign (TAC) in South Africa.

> With just a few paid staffers but a large base of volunteers, TAC won its first victory on this front last November [2000]. The Medical Control Council (MCC), South Africa's drug regulators, granted a first-ever waiver allowing importation of a generic medication for the country's 4 million people with HIV. To accomplish this in a climate in which the government is ambivalent about acknowledging AIDS at all took international activist pressure. But it couldn't have happened without TAC's remarkable squad of HIV positive South Africans. The November success came after a nine-month campaign that included, at one point, the threat of U.S. sanctions and, at another, an offer by five pharmaceuticals to temporarily cut drug prices for southern Africa by 85 percent. TAC welcomed the discounts but condemned any effort to keep the government from promoting importation or manufacture of even cheaper generic substitutes. (Bordowitz, 2001, p. 3)

TAC was closely involved in the demonstrations and activism about treatment access by PWAs and their supporters at the Durban conference. Since 2000 the organization has been successful in mobilizing political action and improving access to treatments. In 2006, for instance, Mark Harrington described the role of TAC in influencing political leadership in South Africa and securing broader access to treatments:

It is too soon to tell how durable and concrete the results of the apparent rapprochement between TAC and the South African government will be. But no one can doubt that the government's turnaround owes an incalculable amount to the unrelenting activism of TAC over the past eight years, and this in turn demonstrates that strong activist movements can transform AIDS policy in countries with functioning democratic institutions. Whether the achievements of TAC can be duplicated in countries which lack full rights for civil society organizations remains to be seen. ... What is needed? More intelligent activism at all levels, such as that illustrated so dramatically by TAC in 2006, is a prerequisite. (Harrington, 2006, p. 5)

Reports on the epidemic around the world, like Harrington's, documented efforts among people with HIV/AIDS to form activist organizations. Not all accounts of expanding AIDS initiatives in developing countries chronicled efforts to gain access to treatments in an African context. Initiatives in many developing countries directed at AIDS prevention, reducing stigma, and meeting the basic needs of communities affected the epidemic were discussed. For instance, in a series of articles chronicling the epidemic in Asia, *POZ magazine* profiled the development of PWA organizations in China, Vietnam, the Philippines, Thailand, Nepal, Sri Lanka and India.

A predominant motif in accounts of community mobilization was emphasizing the leadership of HIV positive organizers and activists. In the case of TAC, after the conference in Durban, Gregg Bordowitz wrote about the influence of Zackie Achmat, Chair of the organization, and his refusal to take medications:

Supporters have offered to purchase HAART meds for Achmat outright, but he's publically declared that he will not take any drugs unless they are available to everyone in South Africa. "I have decided not to take antiretrovirals because I don't want to live in a world that devalues the lives of poor people simply because they are poor. I could never look those people in the eye, and I couldn't lead them, if I was taking my medicines while they were going to die." Achmat's pledge, in the courageous tradition of Ghandi's hunger strikes and Nelson Mandela's refusal to renounce armed struggle to get out of prison, is a display of the kind of leadership that could turn around the AIDS epidemic. In three short years, TAC has not only pushed the South African government to expand HIV drug access, it has helped establish an activist network among poor nations producing, procuring and distributing quality medicines despite trade restrictions and pharmaceutical industry pressure. (Bordowitz, 2001, p. 14)

Individual stories of people with HIV/AIDS who overcame great odds to become activists, like Achmat, were intertwined with descriptions of the organizations or initiatives they were involved in or were integral in starting. Typical is this profile of Russian activist Sergey Myachikov, cofounder of an organization called A.I.D.S.:

> At 24, with a wife and young son, Myachikov has seen quite a bit of "real life." Now, he's one of a small but growing number of Russian activists who are open about having HIV and seek to boost public awareness by talking about their experience. He's determined to make a dent in his homeland's epidemic, which the UN now calls the world's fastest-growing. ... in the past year, Myachikov distributed 3,000 clean syringes as a volunteer for Kolodetz, a group that promotes prevention among drug users. Now he has joined forces with several other positive activists and formed a new public-education organization called A.I.D.S. (All In Danger — Stop). On World AIDS Day, the group carried out its first action, marching around central Moscow with a huge red ribbon and explaining its significance to passers-by — no small feat in a society where HIV, still shrouded in mystery, is so heavily stigmatized. (Tuller, 2003)

Self empowerment and self-determination has been a central tenet in the PWA movement and this ethic was seen to be a crucial component in mobilizing around the crisis in developing nations. As mentioned in the profile of Myachikov, one obstacle to self empowerment in many regions was the fear and stigmatization associated with the disease. Paul Toh, an activist and person with HIV/AIDS in Thailand (cofounder of the Asia Pacific Network for PWAs), describes this issue:

How do you normalize HIV? We have campaigns in Thailand, such as My Positive Life, where we take pictures of healthy people with HIV saying: "I'm a mother living with HIV." "I'm a banker living with HIV," to change people's perception of PWAs. We PWAs have the responsibility to educate the world that we are as normal as you, walking on the street, that I can be your friend and hug you, share a cup with you, and nothing will happen. I won't transmit the disease to you. So much centers around education, especially in developing countries, because lack of information breeds stigmatization. We as infected people have an important role to play in that education, and policy-makers have to recognize that. ... That kind of scenario will protect our rights as positive people, affirm our right to live. We want to be recognized as human beings, not isolated from society and discriminated against. In Thailand, we've begun to cope with this stigmatization; we've been lucky. (Staff, 2001, p. 20)

The obstacles that Toh identifies are reminiscent of efforts (still ongoing) in the PWA movement in North America to normalize HIV/AIDS — to reduce stigma, challenge misconceptions about the disease and enable people with HIV/AIDS to be involved in decisions that affect their lives.

Organizing by people with HIV/AIDS was influenced by the self help movements of the late 1960s. This form of organizing has been criticized for placing too much emphasis on personal self empowerment at the expense of community development and the broader determinants of health. Accounts of organizing by people with HIV/AIDS in developing nations reflect this emphasis on the centrality of personal self empowerment — mobilizing to address the epidemic hinges on those directly affected embracing their HIV status as a form of politicized self identification. An example is the following profile of Carol Nawina Nyirenda:

Carol has lived with HIV for many years and has also survived TB treatment. She has been able to transform this personal experience into a political campaign to address TB/HIV, and has incorporated TB advocacy into her national and global HIV activism. (Treatment Action Group, 2008)

It evident, however, in such profiles that there is attention devoted to highlighting that the conditions and resources need to be in place before people will feel able to publicly disclose their HIV status, organize as a community, and mobilize in response to the epidemic. Activists profiled discuss the challenges posed by broader social determinants like poverty, social justice, employment and infrastructure. In the words of another African activist, Nelson Juma Otwoma from Kenya: "My activism has always been focused on alleviating the burden of poverty and promoting health. I have always had an intense inner feeling that something needed to change" (Treatment Action Group, 2008).

Bridging the Global Gap: The processes of globalization in the PWA movement began in the late 1980s and throughout the 1990s as international networks of people with HIV/AIDS were initiated through community mobilization and the sponsorship of international agencies like the Global AIDS Fund. Whereas Durban was the first International Conference held in Africa, people with HIV/AIDS from around the world had already met in various regions, including Africa in 1995.

> The Global Network of People Living With AIDS/HIV (GNP+) held its 7th International Conference For People With AIDS and HIV in Cape Town, South Africa, March 1995. The theme of the five day conference was "Positive Power To The Global Community," and included workshops and sessions on health, human rights, communication, migration, skills and identities. The conference brought together 800 people with AIDS and HIV from all over the world. It was the first global conference for AIDS held in Africa. The official conference language was English with simultaneous translation into many African, Asian, Latin American and European languages. (Roberts Auli, 1995, p. 1)

Another example of an influential organization initiated in the 1990s is the International Community of Women Living with HIV/AIDS, or ICW:

> The International Community of Women Living with HIV/AIDS (ICW), a registered UK charity, is the only international network run

for and by HIV positive women. ICW was founded in response to the desperate lack of support, information and services available to women living with HIV worldwide and the need for these women to have influence and input on policy development. ICW was formed by a group of HIV positive women from many different countries attending the 8th International Conference on AIDS held in Amsterdam in July 1992. HIV positive women shared stories and strategies for coping and devised action plans for the future. During this meeting, the women agreed that they did not want to lose this momentum and ICW was created. (International Community of Women Living with HIV/AIDS, 2006)

Since the mid 1990s the PWA movement has continued to forge networks across international and global boundaries. The global consciousness emerging the end of the decade, symbolized by the Durban conference, has been a catalyst for further networking among people with HIV/AIDS across developed and developing nations and given momentum to the possibility of a global PWA community.

One of the objectives of networks like GPN+ and ICW is bringing people with HIV/AIDS together from around the world to, in one instance, share their perspectives and worldviews, so as to increase knowledge of the divergent and common challenges posed by the epidemic.

This is a forum of people living with HIV and AIDS in Uganda. It brings together all associations and groups of people living with HIV and AIDS, and our main purpose is to ensure that we have a common voice to fight for our rights, and to ensure that all people living with HIV and AIDS at all levels have been heard and are well represented. It was formed in May 2003 after realization that there was nobody, no organization that was bringing together all associations and networks in the country. (Hemp, 2004, p.19)

This forum, created to bring together organizations in Uganda together, is a good example of a structure designed to unite people with HIV/AIDS across regions so that they can articulate a "common voice" through which to fight for their rights. On another level, such forums and networks have played a more pragmatic role in bringing together people with types of skills and knowledge that can be shared. This exchange of knowledge and skills can be seen in the recent Women's Summit:

> It was the World YWCA, partnering with the International Community of Women Living with HIV/AIDS (ICW), that finally organized this unprecedented women's meeting—known officially as the "International Women's Summit: Women's Leadership Making a Diffference on HIV and AIDS." Kapihya joined leaders from around the world, including hundreds of HIV-positive women, many of them Africans who are emerging as a grassroots force for advocacy on the continent. U.S. pioneers in the movement—such as the positive women of ICW and The Well Project—found the excitement infectious. For many, the Kenya summit was a passing of the torch, as a new generation of women and young girls step up to claim their place as leaders. Nowhere was that more evident than at a day-long, closed-door Positive Women's Forum and a jam-packed public discussion about "Positive Women's Sexual and Reproductive Health Rights." These events were as much celebration as discussion, with whooping African ululation and elaborate clapping giving them the feeling of holy-roller tent revivals. (d'Adesky, 2007, p. 2)

By passing on a shared history, along with skills and knowledge, international networks of people with HIV/AIDS attempt to increase the capacity of individual members and groups from different regions. Yet, on another level, as umbrella advocacy groups, organizations that cut across regions can wield tremendous pressure on governments and international organizations. As one member of the GPN+ noted in a roundtable on the global AID crisis:

> I do see light at the end of the tunnel. Every conference I come to, we bring more and more people in the PWA community together to voice the real issues that we face. And we push governments, policy-makers, UN agencies, to recognize that HIV requires a bottom-up approach. They have to realize that it is the community that moves HIV, not decisions from the top. They need the PWA

community. They need people infected in each community to help them save the world. (Staff, 2001)

The agenda of international organizations is to facilitate the capacity of groups bringing a "bottom up approach" to bear upon the challenges of epidemic in their region by drawing on the knowledge and skills of people with HIV/AIDS around the world. In sharing knowledge and perspective the hope is that the gap between people with HIV/AIDS in developed and developing nations will be lessened.

The actions of international organizations like GPN+ and IWC has raised questions about the possibility and viability of creating a global PWA movement. Accounts of organizing among people with HIV/AIDS post-Durban suggest that there is an increase in political mobilization among people with HIV AIDS. The possibility of a global PWA movement was taken up in forum among activists and published in *POZ magazine*.

Phill: Let's talk about the idea of a global community of people living with AIDS. Can there be such a movement? Alejandra: There already is a global PWA community. We are here, and we have met in different places, or we know each other through magazines or telephone or e-mails. What we need to do is strengthen our community and get more people involved because, as Julian said, it's working — we've really changed the AIDS epidemic. The main issues that join us now are access to treatment, care and love, and the right not to be discriminated against. And we are working in that direction. (Staff, 2001, p. 29)

Among the panel of activists a key issue that emerged was whether it was possible not to create a community as such but to generate a sense of solidarity across the differences that people from different regions bring the HIV/AIDS crisis.

Paul: I agree that there is a global PWA community, but what I'd like to see is global PWA solidarity. I'd like to see all PWAs coming together to fight for a common objective. Once you're infected, it doesn't matter whether you are a gay man or an IV-drug user or a woman — you're just an infected person — and we should understand each other and come together. Especially now, if we are talking about living for many more years — what do we do with our lives? Many of us are still here today because we are lucky to be literate and have resources. People who are infected in the villages, who are illiterate, who have few resources — what about them? They are the same as us, they are positive, and we have a responsibility not to forget them. (Staff, 2001, p. 31)

This participant identifies one of the numerous structural barriers to mobilization among people with HIV/AIDS. In addition to the lack of infrastructure in developing nations, stigma is another factor identified by activists as impeding political action among those infected.

Paul: I don't really see a difference in solidarity in the developed and developing world. If you trace back history, how did ACT UP and all the groups in the developed world achieve what they did? Through solidarity. It was because infected people came together, marched in the streets, changed policies — that's why they got to where they are today. Now this is happening in the developing world, but we have bigger hurdles because we are fighting more stigmatization. We face not just the risk of being HIV positive, but the risk of being killed if we come out openly. (Staff, 2001, p. 42)

The viewpoint that a disease category — HIV/AIDS — can unite individuals and communities with significant differences is a contentious assumption in the PWA movement. In the 1990s in North America, organizing among people with HIV/AIDS struggled with similar issues as the disease affected a more diverse cross section of society. What emerged was a fragmentation of the movement across gender, sexuality, injection drug use and ethnicity. The division between the GPN+ and the IWC suggests that there are divisions — in many respects necessary divisions because of the different needs that people have with regards to their health — within the global PWA movement. The question is whether such divisions serve to weaken the movement or simply make it more diversified.

Emergent Global Issues

The globalization of HIV/AIDS in the late 1990s and after 2000 helped to create new lines of communication between people living with HIV/AIDS across developed and developing regions. A global orientation toward the epidemic raised awareness among people with HIV/AIDS and activists in the United States and Canada about issues and concerns regarding the HIV/AIDS crisis around the world. Representations of the epidemic in PWA publications began to examine in more detail forms of institutional neglect regarding the international response to HIV/AIDS. Reflecting on the year 2000, Mark Milano expressed in the publication *Positively Aware* the sentiment that it was time that those in developed nations begin to pay more attention to the epidemic around the world:

> It's time for people with HIV in the U.S. to realize that as bad as it is for us (and let's not pretend it isn't bad — I lost a number of friends this year), it's incredibly worse for people overseas. And it's not a case of "it's just too big to get a grip on." There are specific things that we can work on here to improve access over there. Urging the drug companies that may be saving your life to stop opposing efforts to save lives in Africa would be a good place to start. (Milano, 2001)

Since the early 1980s those involved in organizing among people with HIV/AIDS exposed forms of institutional neglect and advocated for an increased response to the epidemic among public officials, corporate executives, and health care providers. And while there was an awareness of the epidemic as a global problem throughout the 1990s, the level of involvement and advocacy regarding international neglect and accountability increased after 2000. The primary issue to emerge at this time was increasing global access to treatments for people in Africa and other endemic nations. In addition to treatment access, the centrality of women with HIV/AIDS in the global epidemic was another issue that became apparent with globalization. Lastly, the rise of AIDS denialism on an international level and the resulting stigma related to HIV/AIDS was another key question that emerged with globalization and was identified as a barrier to responding to the pandemic.

Treatment Neglect and Accountability: Advances in treatment and care in the late 1990s improved the lives of many people with HIV/AIDS in developed countries. A central issue in the PWA movement during this time was the importance of ensuring that treatments were affordable and accessible to those most vulnerable. The medical industrial complex — and pharmaceutical corporations primarily — was heavily criticized for misrepresenting their products and profiting unreasonably from the sale of AIDS medications. The emerging globalization of the epidemic in the late 1990s brought into clearer focus the disparities in access to medications between people with HIV/AIDS in developed and developing nations. In November of 1999, John S. James described the situation in Africa regarding access to treatments:

> Over 12,000,000 people in Africa alone have already died of AIDS, and 20,000,000 more in Africa are now living with HIV, according to generally accepted estimates. Worldwide, about 90% of people with HIV live in developing countries and have no access to modern pharmaceuticals, which often cost more than $10,000 per year; the situation is similar for many other serious illnesses including cancer and drug-resistant tuberculosis. (James, 1999, p. 1)

One of the important messages that came from the International AIDS conference in Durban was the realization that it was not only possible but ethically necessary for people with HIV/AIDS to have access to AIDS medications in developing nations. Making this point, the South African activist organization TAC organized a March at the beginning of the conference. Statements made at the march read:

> Anti-retroviral drugs have been shown to extend the lives and improve the health of many people with AIDS and advanced HIV disease. There are drugs that can successfully prevent, treat, and cure the opportunistic infections and co-infections, such as tuberculosis, fungal infections, pneumonias, cancers and malaria that kill most people with HIV and AIDS. People in poor countries

cannot gain access to life-saving medications because of their price. ... Denying people with HIV/AIDS access to affordable medicines in order to protect profits or intellectual property rights is tantamount to genocide. Denying access to treatments or prevention intervention by any government body using the smokescreen of questioning the cause of AIDS is unacceptable. (Treatment Action Campaign, 2000, p. 1)

Greater access to drugs was not only a claim made by PWA organizations and activists. It was a sentiment that quickly gained momentum among delegates at the conference. The contradictions that existed in the means to health among people with HIV/AIDS in developing and developed nations had been made explicit; demands being made to redress the issue were beginning to be taken seriously by governments, drug companies and international agencies.

Pharmaceutical corporations were targeted as the primary institutional barrier to treatment access. With millions of people with HIV/AIDS without treatment in poorer countries, drug companies came under scrutiny for neglecting the needs of the most vulnerable in the world while profiting from the sales of medications. Up until the Durban conference, drug companies were criticized for doing very little and even impeding an international response to the global AIDS epidemic. Discussing the state of global access to treatments, Mark Harrington reviewed initiatives by drug companies prior to 2000:

Until very recently, most companies preferred strategies other than major price reductions for dealing with AIDS in poor countries. These strategies included: (1) ignoring AIDS in the developing world; (2) setting a "one world, one price" policy, in the face of enormous disparities in income between and within countries affected by HIV; (3) selling expensive drugs for AIDS and HIV to tiny rich elites in poor countries; (4) applying pressure on the U.S. and other rich countries to pressure poor countries not to make generic drugs; (5) starting charitable programs in one or a few affected countries to increase support for AIDS-related programs; (6) and most recently, a set of promises to provide developing countries with steep discounts or even free drugs. These most recent

promises were made in the run-up to the Durban AIDS conference
with its inevitable focus on the inaccessibility of treatment for 95%
of the world's 34 million HIV-infected people, and, so far as I am
aware, not one person has received a single pill as a result of any of
these promised price reductions or drug give-away programs.
(Harrington, 2000, section I, p. 3)

Culpability for the lack of treatment options for people with HIV/AIDS in
poorer nations was not placed on pharmaceutical corporations alone.
Harrington's report, like many accounts in PWA publications of
international neglect and accountability, point out that governments in
developed nations and multilateral agencies including UNAIDS (in large
part because of their reliance on the financial support of developed
nations) were slow to respond to the treatment needs of people with
HIV/AIDS in developing nations and did not put pressure on drug
companies to make their medications more accessible (Harrington, 2000).

There were two main strategies for increasing access to treatment to
developing countries that gained prominence around the time of the
Durban conference. One was for drug companies to significantly reduce
the cost of AIDS medications for people with HIV/AIDS in endemic
countries. In 2000, there was considerable activist and public pressure
placed on drug companies to restructure their pricing structure for
HAART medications:

> Shortly before World AIDS Day (December 1), a coalition of AIDS
> and health groups including MSF (Médecins Sans Frontièrs, or
> Doctors Without Borders) called on pharmaceutical companies to
> reduce prices of AIDS drugs 95% in poor countries — reductions
> comparable to those already in use for vaccines and contraceptives.
> … Price reductions up to 85% have already been offered by some
> companies, but even then drug costs approach $1,000 to treat each
> patient for one year — much too expensive for most individuals and
> governments in poor countries. (James, 2000, p. 1)

As John S. James notes, drug companies responded to the call for greater
global accountability on behalf of corporations regarding the health needs
of HIV infected communities in developing countries. Harrington has

documented many of the price reductions that were made in the years after Durban, including instances in which medications were given away:

> In response to a campaign by South Africa's Treatment Action Campaign (TAC) and Médecins sans Frontières (MSF), Pfizer has agreed to provide free fluconazole (Diflucan) to South Africans who are diagnosed with cryptococcal meningitis. However, this offer is restricted to one country and one AIDS complication. TAC and MSF have demanded that Pfizer broaden the offer to include treatment for esophageal candidiasis and to include other poor countries, or that Pfizer agree to a compulsory license for a local company to manufacture cheap generic fluconazole. (Harrington, 2000)

Pharmaceutical corporations provided relief not only in the form of price reductions and discounts. Hoffmann-La Roche and Merck contributed funds under infrastructure and health care programs supported by UNAIDS, the Global AIDS Fund and the Gates Foundation. Bristol-Myers Squibb financed their own projects in Africa to facilitate AIDS prevention, treatment and research programs (Harrington, 2000). Yet, as Harrington points out, none of the initiatives by drug companies came close to being sufficient in redressing the need for treatments: "Whatever the fate of differential pricing, in any case, the programs announced to date will reduce prices too little and reach too few of the world's HIV infected people" (Harrington, 2000).

Recognizing that reductions in the prices of drugs was not a viable solution, people with HIV/AIDS and activists writing in PWA publications embraced a second strategy to increase access to treatments by making generic medications more available to those infected in poorer nations. One of the main barriers to the use of generic medications is the patents that pharmaceutical corporations hold, John S. James explains:

> About 90% of people with HIV live in developing countries and have no access to modern medicines even when necessary to save their lives — in part because new drugs are usually patented for 20 years and priced for the developed world. When generic copies are

available, they often sell for a small fraction of the price; some essential medicines could be sold at a profit for a tenth of their current prices, and be available to millions of people now denied them. The patent holders are multinational pharmaceutical companies, who have little interest anyway in marketing their drugs in poor countries — but the industry is intensely interested in preventing any precedents which might threaten major markets in the U.S., Europe, or elsewhere. (James, 1999, p. 2)

Treatment advocates consistently pointed out that without the market protection actions of drug companies and developed nations, access to medications could be expanded tremendously. This point is made by Mark Milano — a member of ACT/UP New York — in his report from the Durban conference when the issue of generic medications took root:

> Durban also saw the beginning of a new hope: the realization that treatment was a possibility for poor nations, if the drug companies and the U.S. government would stop fighting their legal efforts to produce generic versions of lifesaving meds. I joined a group of activists that hounded candidate Al Gore until he pressured the U.S. Trade Representative to change trade policies regarding nations that produce generic drugs without the permission of the patent holder. ... Our work did lead generic manufacturers to finally reveal what we had suspected for years: that a three-drug combo could be produced in large quantities for less than $300 a year! That's right — the same drugs we pay over $12,000 for could be made available to poor nations for a fraction of what we're charged for them. (Milano, 2001, p. 11)

Accompanying the push to make generic drugs more available was the idea that developing nations should be allowed to manufacture and distribute their own AIDS medications. In the late 1990s, the Brazilian government led this charge by manufacturing generic HIV/AIDS treatments and distributing them for free to people with HIV/AIDS.

Of all the developing countries, Brazil has done the best job of making anti-HIV treatment available to a significant proportion of its 580,000 HIV-infected people. Since Brazil never had restrictive patent laws which limit the use of generic drugs in, for example, South Africa or Guatemala, it started making its own nucleoside analogues ... in the mid-1990s. Brazil invoked the "national emergency" provisions of the Trade Related Intellectual Property (TRIPs) clause of the WTO treaty to begin manufacturing its own antiretrovirals. (Harrington, 2000)

Brazil has been held up as leading the movement among developing nations toward producing generic drugs and making them accessible to people with HIV/AIDS. After Durban, a number of countries, including Thailand, have followed Brazil in challenging international patent legislation by producing their own medications. Since 2000, pharmaceutical corporations have been portrayed as reluctantly conceding the right of developing countries to declare HIV/AIDS a national emergency enabling them to create their own generic medications. It may be only a matter of time before drug companies begin to take action against countries that are perceived to be breaking patents laws, as in the case of Abbot Laboratories and the Thailand government (Staff, 2007).

Despite the recognition that access to medications was important, some activists and people with HIV/AIDS argued that infrastructure development and broader determinants of health should be greater priorities for developing nations. At the International Conference in Barcelona in 2002 the question of treatment versus prevention and capacity building emerged as a central concern especially with the availability of funds through UNAIDS and the Global AIDS Fund.

Prevention gives more bang for the buck, the researchers argued, as evidenced by interventions in Uganda and Thailand, where infection trends had been reversed — and where there was no risk that half-assed HAART would spawn a drug-resistant supervirus. "What about the 40 million already infected?" the treatment-access camp shot back. Pointing to Brazil's lauded universal-treatment model, which proves cost-effective by preventing recurrent hospitalizations, the advocates argued that treating wasn't just the right thing, but the smart thing. At that day's plenary, the temporary last word in the escalating debate on treatment access was had by drugs-into-bodies advocates. Their voices eclipsed the naysayers, the proponents of "infrastructure first." ... Graca Machel thundered that the moral imperative to treat transcends cost-effectiveness: "On a continent with 28 million people living with HIV, there are only 30,000 people receiving [HIV meds]. How can we hear these figures and still be having discussions on patents and how not to lose money?" (Feuer, 2002, p. 17)

In this report from the conference, Cindra Feuer summarized the debate between the two approaches to development and aid. While couched in terms of development, many treatment activists — especially people with HIV/AIDS in developing countries — perceived the infrastructure argument as an attempt by drug companies, governments and those in positions of power to exert control over the market for medications by discrediting the "drugs into bodies" advocates. While this debate continued beyond Barcelona, increasingly it became evident that an ethical and effective international response needed to address both sides of this dilemma: treatment access and infrastructure development.

Global Epidemic among Women with HIV/AIDS: Since the beginning of the epidemic the needs of women with HIV/AIDS have been, if not ignored outright, kept in the background of the epidemic. In response, organizations by and for women with HIV/AIDS formed so as to fill the gap in existing AIDS support, treatment, advocacy and prevention. Women Alive, for instance, is a national organization formed in 1991 by and for people with HIV/AIDS that, through a range of services and programs, seeks to

set the standard of quality care for women with HIV/AIDS ... challenge national policies on treatment and prevention of HIV/AIDS ... provide community leadership and mentor other women to become effective advocates ... combat stigma and eliminates isolation, generate treatment research for women with HIV infection... and make HIV information reachable and understandable to every woman throughout the world. (Women Alive, 2009)

Coalitions like Women Alive have been influential in highlighting forms of institutional neglect toward women with HIV/AIDS, like the exclusion of women from clinical trials and the media contributing to the myth of HIV as a gay male disease. And, while it was necessary and continues to be necessary for women with HIV/AIDS to struggle for the right to health, in the 1990s the work of organizations like Women Alive increased awareness about the gender dimensions of the HIV/AIDS epidemic. Despite the momentum created by activists and women with HIV/AIDS in the 1990s, the predominate view of HIV/AIDS, as least from a North American perspective, was that it remains an epidemic most prominent among men.

The globalization of HIV/AIDS in the late 1990s raised awareness about the extent to which women are at the centre of the global pandemic. In Durban at the International AIDS Conference in 2000 the needs and interests of women with HIV/AIDS were brought to the attention of institutional authorities and the public in developing and developed nations. Project Inform reported on this component of the conference as follows:

> Globally, women and girls comprise the growing majority of people living with HIV. Reflecting this shift in the epidemic was an increased focus on women's issues at the 13th International Conference on AIDS. In all of its sessions, the conference grappled with many of the issues facing women and girls living with, and at risk for, HIV. Appropriately, many of the discussions focused on the plight of women in sub-Saharan Africa and other resource-poor areas. Nearly all sessions highlighted the inequities in human rights, HIV care and resources between sexes, classes and nations. ... The conference did break ground by providing attendees with a clear understanding of just how much this disease impacts women in the developing world. Moreover, it left attendees with a better sense of the difficult work that lies ahead and a renewed desire to undertake that work. (Project Inform, 2000, p. 1)

Leading up to Durban, grassroots efforts among women globally had gained momentum throughout the 1990s. Transnational networks like the

International Community of Women Living with HIV/AIDS and the Global Network of People with HIV/AIDS brought women with HIV/AIDS together in meetings and conferences so that they might organize a stronger community based response to the epidemic. Reflecting on Durban, Yvette Delph recalls the importance of groundwork done at previous conferences organized by and for women in the 1990s:

> I would also like to draw the analogy between ... attending Durban this year and attending the Beijing Women's Conference in 1995. ...I think that five years later we've seen that what it has meant is that grassroots women and organizations have come together, that they have proliferated, that they have met with greater understanding of their basic rights from the people — whether as women or rights in terms of reproduction. It has meant that there is pressure on governments to ensure that people know these rights, that these rights are enshrined in legislation and in practice. There has been a tremendous pressure, for example, to address issues of bride burning, of female genital mutilation, all kinds of things. And it has brought both to the fore as issues and the pressure has been maintained, and I think that progress has been made. I don't think enough progress has been made ... but at the same time, I would not want to minimize the impact that those conferences have had. (Treatment Action Group, 2000, p. 27-30)

After years of working toward raising gender as a key issue with regards to the HIV/AIDS epidemic, awareness of the severity of the global AIDS crisis in developing countries brought into focus the spread of the epidemic among women. The globalization of HIV/AIDS helped to make clear that an international response to the epidemic needed to be organized around addressing the needs and interests of women with HIV/AIDS.

At the Durban conference a number of issues were raised with regards to the needs and rights of women with HIV/AIDS. Little advancement had been made in the area of treatment and care for women. Instead the highlight was on the spread of infection among women and the need for better prevention strategies. At the forefront of prevention was reproduction and more specifically mother to child transmission:

One of the most important themes at the International AIDS Conference in Durban was the prevention of mother-to-child transmission of HIV (MTCT). This was very appropriate given that one in four South African women in their peak child-bearing years — between the ages of 20 and 29 — are HIV-positive. In addition, rates of HIV infection in prenatal clinics in sub-Saharan Africa can run as high as 43%. While progress to reduce the rates of MTCT continues to move steadily forward, the conference highlighted the global disparities between developed and developing countries in implementing such interventions. (Cadman & Kaminski, 2000, p. 1)

As pointed out in this account, with the prevalence of HIV increasing in developing countries, ensuring that women with HIV/AIDS have access to medications would decrease mother to child transmission. Unfortunately, the lack of political will and the availability of resources were identified by activists and people with HIV/AIDS as ongoing barriers to this form of prevention. In 2003, John S. James reported in *AIDS Treatment News* that

about 800,000 children are infected with HIV each year through mother-to-child transmission, and hundreds of thousands of these cases could be prevented. Cost of the nevirapine is not the problem. The main obstacle has been funding and implementing the programs to use it (which usually require testing, counseling, dealing with stigma such as violence against women who test positive, staff training, prenatal care, and associated infrastructure). Only about 1% of Africans now have access to services for prevention of mother-to-child transmission of HIV, according to a World Health Organization report issued September 1, 2003. (James, 2003, p. 4)

Consistent with the emphasis on treatment activism at Durban and afterward, the debate regarding mother to child transmission concentrated primarily on access to medications. A prominent view was that women needed to first have access to treatments before broader social and political barriers, like stigma, could be addressed. Supporting this approach, women with HIV/AIDS from developing nations claimed they were more open to having their families tested if medications were available (Freuer, 2002). There were accounts in PWA publications, however, that countered this approach by arguing that more attention needed to be placed on the broader determinants to health or the means to health for women. Activists and women with HIV/AIDS were also critical of the emphasis placed on reproduction — and control over reproduction — as the central concern regarding women and HIV/AIDS among public officials, scientists, and health care professionals.

Despite the tendency toward medicalizing the needs of women with HIV/AIDS, the significance of Durban remained that women and girls could no longer be sidelined in the institutional and international response to the global AIDS epidemic. Instead, the needs and interests of women with HIV/AIDS in developing nations came to be seen as the focal point in AIDS prevention on a global scale. Furthermore, the issue of mother to child transmission pointed to the linkages between treatment and prevention initiatives. As shown in this overview of the meetings in Barcelona in 2002, women with HIV/AIDS continued to be a central concern after Durban:

> Women were very visible in the political discussion at the conference. As the numbers of women and girls infected continue to rise at alarming rates, women and men are struggling to address issues for positive women, including the gender inequities that fuel the epidemic. A woman with HIV opened the conference and an HIV-positive woman closed the conference with an eloquent and compelling speech urging, among many things, a greater role for community at the next conference in Bangkok. Women at high levels of government and in leadership positions spoke about their own actions, the concept of leadership, what was needed for women living with HIV and the importance of gender equality. (Project Inform, 2003, p. 19)

Activists and people with HIV/AIDS made efforts to keep the needs and interests of women at the forefront of AIDS treatment and prevention in developing nations. This work included advocating for more scientific research that is clinically relevant to women along with social, political and economic infrastructure development that includes communities of women infected and affected by HIV/AIDS. While sexism and racism continued to be significant barriers in the response to HIV/AIDS, globalization had helped to put gender equity on the list of infrastructural development that was necessary to alleviate the gap in resources between developing and developed nations.

AIDS Dissidents and Denialism: As a medical condition, HIV/AIDS has been contested by a small number of scientists, activists and people diagnosed with the illness who call into question the scientific legitimacy of the syndrome and the epidemic. This skepticism about the connection between HIV and AIDS has taken several forms over the last twenty five years. Early in the epidemic, scientists Peter Duesberg and David Rasnick contested the diagnostic category of AIDS as a single disease entity; instead, the illnesses experienced by those diagnosed may not be necessary linked, be connected to the immune system, or have a single cause (the HIV virus) (Mirken, 2000). In publications by and for people living with HIV/AIDS those identified as dissidents are occasionally given opportunities to voice their views but are more routinely reprimanded for propagating dangerous misinformation about the disease.

> Members of these groups have claimed that the AIDS epidemic is over — if indeed it ever existed — and that the world would be better off if people stopped using protease inhibitors and other HIV medications. Disagree with them and run the risk of being shouted down, intimidated and driven out of the group. With the original ACT UP mission destroyed and abandoned, long-term members have been forced to move along, regroup or mutate into other organizations. (Salyer, 2000, p. 6)

Like in this critique by David Salyer in *Survival News*, AIDS dissidents have also been taken to task for discrediting and reversing the organizing done by activists and people with HIV/AIDS in response to the epidemic. With advancements in treatment options, those involved in organizations like Health Education AIDS Liaison (HEAL) have publicly claimed that a positive HIV test does not lead to AIDS. Dissidents or denialists, as they are often referred, warn that taking toxic HIV medications like HAART causes illnesses among otherwise healthy people mistakenly diagnosed with HIV or AIDS.

In the late 1999s momentum behind the relatively small dissident movement increased when South African President Thabo Mbeki began to seek the expertise of individuals associated with the AIDS dissident movement in anticipation of the International AIDS conference in Durban. Accounts from the conference claim that Mbeki sought to assemble a group of experts — denialists and nondissidents — that could provide insight into the problem of HIV/AIDS in Africa. In his article on the conference, and participation in the forum (as a non-denialist), David Scondras wrote:

> As I sat in Kingsmead Cricket Stadium waiting for the conference's opening ceremony to begin, in a city on the warm waters of the Indian Ocean, with roads better paved than in my Boston home, surf-boarders, Internet cafés and fine restaurants, my thoughts floated back to the letter I'd received this spring. It was from President Thabo Mbeki, inviting me, as head of the HIV-treatment advocacy group Search for a Cure, to join his advisory panel on AIDS. Besides asking us to address the notorious question of whether HIV causes AIDS, Mbeki challenged us to determine why the disease attacks such different populations in his country and in the North, and what responses make sense given South Africa's economic realities. The panel was to meet twice and submit a report before the Durban conference. (Wright et al., 2000)

Unsure as to whether to participate — fearing that his involvement might give legitimacy to the denialist perspective — Scondras described the debate that ensued between denialists and nondenialists about what advice should be given to government officials in South Africa.

> At the second meeting — another parallel-universe talkfest — Mbeki was presented with two options: We round-earthers recommended using antiretrovirals in late-stage illness, offering nevirapine to prevent mother-to-child transmission, treating STDs and other possible AIDS cofactors, and improving nutrition and public health. The denialists urged not treating HIV, but rather

reducing drug addiction and such "immune stressors" as malnutrition. The best way to end the epidemic, said David Rasnick, MD, of the University of California at Berkeley, would be to "get rid of the HIV test." (Wright et al., 2000)

The reaction to the involvement of AIDS denialists in policy development prior to the conference was swift and decisive. There were calls made by scientists and government officials to boycott the conference. At the International Conference, a group of scientists and physicians wrote the Durban Declaration refuting many of the claims made by denialists and affirming that HIV causes AIDS.

The controversy caused by Mbeki's involvement of AIDS denialists at the International conference in Durban was significant in that it drew attention to the ideological barriers that exist in many developing nations with regard to HIV/AIDS. On one level, activists and people with HIV/AIDS pointed out that attending to skepticism about whether HIV is the cause of AIDS served as an unfortunate distraction from developing effective treatment and prevention initiatives.

Despite its weaknesses and unsolved problems, AIDS research is continuing to make progress against the disease. The far bigger task before us today, perhaps, is to overcome the economic and social barriers that prevent progress from being available to all those living with HIV. Despite the early perceptions that the Durban conference would disintegrate into a shouting match between AIDS specialists and a tiny worldwide group of so-called "AIDS denialists," once the conference opened the collective wisdom of all those who contributed to it prevailed. The spotlight of world attention was turned away from a few disturbing characters pursuing their own publicity and instead focused on the devastating need for care, treatment, prevention, increased human rights and public health infrastructure for millions of people in developing countries now living with HIV. (Project Inform, 2000, p. 10)

In this review of the conference in *Perspectives*, a publication of the treatment organization Project Inform, the message, widely stated after Durban, was that endorsing or embracing denialist claims impeded the formulation of an international response to HIV/AIDS. Activists and people with HIV/AIDS from developing nations, similarly, were concerned about the use of this perspective by government officials to slow or block treatment or prevention efforts.

> While the scientific tug-of-war proceeds, those whose lives are directly affected are becoming frustrated. PWA Zackie Achmat, a cofounder of the South African Treatment Action Campaign, grants that the panel could be beneficial if it raised the AIDS ed levels of the population, which he describes as "scientifically illiterate." And he acknowledges that "it is crucial that the government gets the information it needs to move forward," especially since "we have a very different scale of the epidemic in South Africa than in the developed world." But his ultimate message about Mbeki's action is one of concern: "The debates around the causality of AIDS and the toxicity of antiretrovirals are obscuring the real issue: drug-pricing policies that have left many essential meds unaffordable for the vast majority of South Africans with HIV. Rather than waste precious time reopening dead debates, the government should commit sufficient resources to addressing this crisis." (Cullinan & Thom, 2000)

The views expressed by Achmat were accompanied by a broader concern among activists and people with HIV/AIDS in developing and developed nations that the proliferation of denialist claims would deepen rather than refute the stigma associated with the disease in endemic countries. This concern was exacerbated by the brutal death of two HIV positive South African people with HIV/AIDS prior to the conference:

> Extreme examples of the social consequences of the stigma against HIV in South Africa include the murders of Mpho Motloung and Gugu Dlamini. Ms. Motloung was murdered by her husband when both went for their HIV test results. Ms. Dlamini, an openly HIV-positive advocate, was stoned to death by a mob. Fear and ignorance are the catalysts for such brutal behavior. This situation is exacerbated by the continuous message coming through in both the media and the government prevention campaign that HIV is a death

sentence, a view strongly opposed by TAC. Not only has this message resulted in much misery (and abuse of women as in the Motloung and Dlamini cases), but it also discourages people from having HIV tests or disclosing their HIV status. It also undermines prevention because people with HIV are discriminated against and believe their situation is hopeless. (Geffen, 2000, p. 21)

The globalization of HIV/AIDS post Durban brought to light the problem of stigma regarding HIV/AIDS in developing nations. In many developing nations, the normalization of HIV/AIDS, fueled by the availability of treatments, meant that the stigma surround the disease has been reduced (though certainty not eliminated). The proliferation of denialist viewpoints in places like South Africa made it evident that work needed to be done to educate those in developing nations — both institutional authorities and the general public — about HIV/AIDS. Activist groups like TAC in South Africa have begun to raise public awareness about HIV/AIDS in an attempt to reduce stigma. While the views and influence of AIDS dissidents and denialists have not gained credibility internationally in the years following Durban, the problem of stigma and the denial — especially among government officials — of either the existence of HIV/AIDS or its prevalence has continued to be identified by activists and people with HIV/AIDS as a significant barrier to addressing the epidemic globally.

Conclusion

In the late 1990s, the conditions for globalization arising over the last thirty years changed the way HIV/AIDS is conceptualized in North America. Economic interdependence between developing and developed nations — especially the reliance of global capitalism on the availability of cheap labour for manufacturing — meant that the health and well-being of those who produce and those who consume are intertwined and made visible by the global mass media, in ways previously unimagined. Multinational corporations, like pharmaceutical industries, not bound by any single governmental policy or regulation, have expanded their scope to include developing nations as emerging markets for products and services. As Raymond Smith notes in his article on Africa in *Body Positive*, the mobility of people globally has brought people across nations together more frequently and in greater numbers than ever before:

> The microlinkages that bind people together in everyday life are well known to us from our own experience. Much less intuitive, however, are the macrolinkages that can bridge different continents and distinct populations of people. Immigration is an obvious source of population transfer, but in a globalized world, other forces interconnecting such seemingly separate communities — and separate epidemics — can be surprisingly powerful. Consider three of the most important: mass tourism, work migration, and refugee displacement. ... Taken together [they] ... account for a good deal of the world's exchange of people — and of HIV. (Smith, 2001 , p. 22)

In a "globalized world" the spread of HIV/AIDS in developing nations and the resulting devastation became increasingly difficult to ignore in the developed world. Activists and people with HIV/AIDS began to formulate strategies for reaching out to communities in developed nations and pressuring governments and international agencies to do more in addressing the crisis expanding in endemic countries since the late 1980s. Nonetheless, not until the International AIDS conference in Durban did institutional authorities in developed countries realize the extent of the crisis in Africa and Asia and that they could and needed to have a role in responding to the overlapping global epidemics around the world.

Between 2000 and 2006 activists and people with HIV/AIDS used PWA publications to comment on and track key themes in the global response to the pandemic. This commentary was an extension of prior efforts in the 1990s to track and raise awareness about the spread of HIV/AIDS in developing nations around the world. In this chapter I examined the portrayal of three prominent issues that emerged post Durban regarding the global pandemic: access to treatments; women and HIV; and AIDS denial and stigma. Interestingly, growing awareness of the pandemic in developing nations was a catalyst for looking at more closely at similar issues developed nations, in this instance North America. As with globalization, the process of becoming interdependent across social, political and geographic boundaries transforms our relationship both globally and locally. A primary concern among activists and people with HIV/AIDS was increasing global access to AIDS medications. Still, the irony of portraying HAART as "life saving" in poorer countries, yet problematic in terms of resistance and side effects in developed counties did not go unnoticed. One review of the International AIDS Conference in Bangkok was entitled: "How to Get 6 Million Poor People on Antiretroviral Therapy — and 1 Million Rich People Off."

In a July editorial, "Freedom of Choice," UK-based AIDS Treatment Update editor Edwin Bernard captures the essence of the present day therapeutic conundrum. "It's ironic," he writes, "that whilst the main focus of this summer's XV International AIDS Conference in Bangkok was on finding ways to get everyone who needs therapy onto HAART, treatment interruption has become a hot topic in well-resourced countries, as concerns over resistance and side effects are increasingly recognized as issues in managing HIV disease" (Treatment Action Group, 2004, p. 1).

Contrasting the developed versus developing response to treatments served to highlight the complexity of the issue and the realization that there are not simple solutions to AIDS treatment and prevention initiatives. The debate between access to treatments versus political and economic infrastructure development continue unresolved in both developed and developing nations. In the case of gender, awareness of the spread of HIV/AIDS among women and girls in developing nations helped to draw attention to this issue locally. For instance, this discussion of women and HIV in a global context included an account of the local state of affairs regarding gender:

At the XV International AIDS Conference in Bangkok there was significant focus on the greater vulnerability of women, particularly young women, to HIV disease. Evidence of their greater risk is demonstrated by the ever increasing body count of infected women nearly everywhere in the world one looks. This evidence didn't appear overnight. The numbers of infected women have been increasing in ever greater and disproportionate numbers for the last 20 years. ... When it comes to ever increasing numbers of women being infected even Wyoming mirrors global trends. The number of women infected in Wyoming has gone from 13% of HIV cases for the years 1989 through 1993 to 37% of cases for 1999 through 2003. Around the world, young people (15-24) make up 50% of the 8,000 new HIV infections occurring daily. (Palmer, 2004, p. 3)

After decades of being overlooked and neglected in a developed context, concern about the spread of HIV/AIDS among women and girls in endemic countries was a catalyst for looking at the lives of women with HIV/AIDS and women at risk in developed nations. A similar situation occurred with regards to AIDS dissidents and denialism. The controversy surrounding the influence of those identified as AIDS dissidents prior to and during the International AIDS Conference in Durban contributed to a greater awareness of organizations in a North American context that question the relationship between HIV and AIDS. There was concern, as shown this article in POZ Magazine, that with a diminished AIDS movement in North America, the mobilization of those who deny the existence of HIV could have serious repercussions for AIDS programs.

But this is also a group that, at a time when AIDS militancy has largely vanished, has rallied like-minded allies in a number of cities to start new chapters. In the past year, dissident ACT UPs have sprung up in Toronto, Atlanta and Hollywood. (In addition to Survive AIDS and Philadelphia, the most prominent "traditional" or "true" ACT UP chapters are Los Angeles, Boston, East Bay [California], New York, Washington, DC, and Paris.) In June, the four dissident ACT UPs took out a full page in Roll Call, the daily paper of Capitol Hill, calling upon legislators to end federal AIDS funding. (Szymanski, 2000, p. 8)

The threat of AIDS denialism led many writers and commentators revisit the debates in PWA publications. John S. James featured a series of articles on denialists in 2001 in order to revisit and support the credibility behind the scientific medicine underlying HIV and AIDS and the consequences of questioning the existence of this disease: "Our concern is not the ideas ... but rather the direct translation of casual speculation and debating points into the medical care of patients with life-threatening illness" (James, 2001, p. 3). This concern with denialists also speaks to the continued problem of stigma associated with HIV/AIDS in both developing and developed nations.

Accounts of the epidemic by activists and people with HIV/AIDS during this period of globalization raised many issues beyond gender, treatment access and denialists. Topics beyond the scope of this chapter include the need to redefine HIV/AIDS as an issue of human rights and social and political security; the rise and fall of the global AIDS fund and international agencies formed post Durban to fund treatment and prevention initiatives in developing nations; the central place of government leadership in building infrastructure and developing policies that address the needs and interests of those most vulnerable. Attention to such issues in developing nations also served to raise awareness of the dwindling institutional response to the epidemic in North America.

> The truth is that the United States ranks among the poor and developing countries today in its response to AIDS by almost any measure: One out of every seven African American men living in DC are infected with HIV, a statistic that measures up with the worst countries in southern Africa. More than 250,000 people in the United States today who are in need of anti-retroviral drugs don't have access. Nearly fifty percent of Black men who have sex with men in this country are infected, but we lack the political will to do anything about it. (King, 2007, p. 34)

Looking at accounts of the epidemic in PWA publications it is evident that the trend toward globalization had served to revitalize mobilization and activism among people with HIV/AIDS in developing nations. In many countries in which in the epidemic is endemic, communities of people living with HIV/AIDS have come together in order to become involved in the decisions that affect their lives and work toward achieving health from below. One of the key questions that this revitalization poses is whether this trend will spark a repoliticalization of the PWA movement in developed nations. In 2006 POZ Magazine ran an article identifying people who could potentially help to reanimate the movement:

In this post-protease climate of AIDS complacency, it sometimes seems that the ferocity exhibited by early activists and advocates has been forgotten. If this 25th anniversary year of the pandemic has shown us anything, it's the dire need for new heroes and heroines to ante up the fight. Fortunately for those of us fending for our lives and those whose lives can perhaps be saved through prevention tactics, POZ has discovered a renewed vigor in global anti-AIDS efforts. (Villarosa et al., 2006)

The possibility of a renewed global PWA movement will hinge upon issues that have historically posed a challenge to political organizing around disease categories like HIV/AIDS. People with HIV/AIDS, through their involvement in local, national and global networks, will need to find common interests and solidarity that transcend social forces that create difference whether based on gender, politics, religion or geography.

CONCLUSION

This book traces the development of organizing and activism by people with HIV/AIDS across four key phases of the epidemic in North America. Writing and publishing by people living with HIV/AIDS trace contours of what it has meant to live, survive and thrive collectively in the context of a health crisis. From the initial formation of the PWA movement, through the normalization of HIV/AIDS in the public sphere, to developments in treatment and most recently the increasing globalization, people with HIV/AIDS have created and used counter public forums to engage in the struggle over the representation and misrepresentation of the pandemic. To close, I describe highlights from the most recent International AIDS Conference in Mexico in 2008. The announcement that under ideal circumstances, people with HIV/AIDS may be noninfectious precipitated a response, the Mexico Manifesto, from PWA organizations. The Manifesto outlined their position on this announcement and its potential ramifications for people with HIV/AIDS. Though it is too early to tell, as in prior years the articulation of this manifesto may indicate a shift in PWA organizing and activism. Certainly, there are signs of a renewed commitment to self-empowerment and community development. Long-standing challenges facing people with HIV/AIDS, often portrayed in institutional discourses as over, are back on the agenda. People with HIV/AIDS are writing about the current problem of stigma and the increasing threat of criminalization, as they did in the 1980s. Another ongoing challenge is the need to sustain solidarity across the diversity of people with HIV/AIDS while acknowledging the different needs and interests in the HIV/AIDS community. Furthermore, the difficulties associated with advancements in AIDS treatment and care, often overlooked in institutional discourses, are addressed as forms of institutional neglect that needs to be rectified. This dialogue about treatment often emphasizes access, not only globally but also in local impoverished communities.

XVII International AIDS Conference: The Mexico Manifesto

In January of 2008, the Swiss Federal Commission for HIV/AIDS announced findings from a study indicating that a person with HIV/AIDS could be noninfectious under ideal circumstances, meaning they are adherent to their medications under the care of a physician, did not have other sexually transmitted infections, and had an undetectable viral load for six months (Bernard, 2008). At first, this news did not receive widespread attention from people with HIV/AIDS, AIDS workers, or institutional authorities. Yet, by the beginning of the International AIDS Conference in Mexico in August, the evidence put forward that people with HIV/AIDS under specific circumstances could be noninfectious became a point of contention among delegates and participants. In his report on the conference, Menadue (2008, p.7) describes a session in which Swiss scientists qualify their announcement:

> In a satellite session the statement was debated. Investigator Professor Pietro Vernazza from the Swiss Federal AIDS Commission who authored the statement said that it was not their intention to say that there was no risk to people having sex with an HIV-positive individual but it was up to the individual to decide if that risk was within the risks they would take in every day life. The best person able to make this decision was a steady partner of an HIV-positive individual who could assess their partner's adherence to antiretrovirals and regular viral load monitoring.

In a number of sessions at the conference, delegates expressed concerns that the findings from the Commission's study might be misunderstood and lead to the perception that people with HIV/AIDS did not have to take precautions to prevent the spread of HIV through unprotected sex or sharing needles. The Associate Director of Strategic Information and Chief Scientific Officer at UNAIDS noted a case in which sex workers had interpreted the announcement as meaning that they no longer needed to use condoms when having sex with clients (Bernard, 2008). The message from delegates concerned about the implications of findings was that this may change prevention strategies for a small number of those HIV positive individuals who fall under the specific criteria; however, for most people with HIV/AIDS around the world the possibility of non-infectiousness is not realistic and potentially misleading. In the article by Bernard (2008), the UNAIDS Associate Director of Strategic Information and Chief Scientific Officer is quoted as saying "we have to be very careful about what we are saying and to whom it applies, because it can have unintended, negative consequences."

At a summit for people with HIV/AIDS held prior to the International conference, participants widely discussed and debated the Swiss declaration. The pre-conference sought to "strengthen the PLHIV movement through promoting the involvement and leadership of people living with HIV in the global HIV response, as well as to enhance PLHIV participation and programming at both the Positive Leadership Summit and AIDS 2008" (Menadue, 2008, p.1). According to Menadue's (2008) account of the meetings, the list of topics under discussion included: "universal access to HIV treatment, care and prevention programmes; positive Prevention (PP); sexual and reproductive rights; criminalisation of HIV transmission; women and most at-risk groups" (p. 5). In sessions, participants debated the implications of non-infectiousness for the already complex set of factors that shape "positive prevention." The summit set the stage for writing a "call to action" by people with HIV/AIDS about the Swiss declaration — titled the Mexico Manifesto — to be presented at the at the International AIDS Conference. The Manifesto begins,

A Call to Action by People with HIV and AIDS presented at the XVII International AIDS Conference 2008, Mexico City. The publication on January 30th 2008 of the Swiss Federal HIV/AIDS Committee (EKAF) in "Schweizerische Ärztezeitung," concerning the non-infectiousness of people with HIV has caused quite a stir. The resulting debate about the evidence and studies on which the

EKAF declaration is based, and the criticism concerning the broad publication of such knowledge, has mobilised the organisations of people living with HIV and their representatives. (LHIVE, 2008)

The document encouraged public officials and health care professionals to recognize the EKAF declaration and revise their perspectives on people with HIV/AIDS and current approaches to AIDS prevention, treatment and care. Any attempt to limit access to information about the EKAF declaration for fear of it misleading people or misdirecting prevention efforts is a form of censorship and portrays people with HIV/AIDS as unable to make their own informed decisions. As Strub (2008) noted in his address to the 2008 United States Conference on AIDS, there are concerns that officials might suppress the findings from the EKAF for fear that they could subvert current prevention strategies:

> The provocative Swiss statement was first met by silence or outright rejection from most AIDS policy leaders in the United States, who were more intent on reinforcing the "use a condom every time" message than taking advantage of an extraordinary opportunity to engage the community in a more nuanced discussion about risk reduction, and the impact of antiretroviral treatment on infectiousness.

Authors of the manifesto called for the accurate representation of people with HIV/AIDS and for prevention and treatment strategies that recognized social inequalities and relied on social integration over exclusion or criminalization. Portrayals of people with HIV/AIDS have historically relied on images of contagion, risk, fear, and irresponsibility. Since the beginning of the epidemic, those living with the disease have called for the right to live sexual and intimate lives; that the response to HIV/AIDS needed to stress social inclusion and acceptance. This sentiment is echoed by Strub:

> "Put simply, the sexuality of people with HIV is considered more as a threat to society than it is as a fundamental and necessary part of our lives and identity. Our right to intimacy has been devalued,

despite the Denver Principles" proclamation of "as full and satisfying sexual and emotional lives as anyone else." Restoring complete intimacy to the sexual lives of people with HIV is of vital importance to the dignity, quality of life and health of people with HIV. Moreover, social integration, without the crippling burdens of stigma or stereotyping, is crucial to reducing the spread of the virus and enabling people with HIV to fulfill one of the responsibilities outlined in the Denver Principles, which is to disclose their HIV status to their sex partners (Strub, 2008).

In Strub's speech, he expresses the intent in the Manifesto to use the EKAF declaration as a vehicle for discussing the real lives of people with HIV/AIDS and redressing the historical legacy of misrepresentation that has mired official response to the health crisis. At the end of the manifesto, the authors argued that the global response to the epidemic needed to more closely link prevention and access to treatments. Since the Durban Conference in 2000, there has been a growing momentum to tie access to treatment with prevention efforts globally. The EKAF declaration moved the debate further by providing evidence that treatment could lead to prevention. Again, echoing the manifesto, Strub (2008) makes that point that "nearly everyone agreed that the Swiss statement had begun the vitally important process of understanding the effect of treatment on prevention."

PWA Self-Empowerment: Emerging Themes

The EKAF declaration and the Mexico Manifesto were high points for PWA self empowerment at the International Conference in 2008. However, discussions in sessions and panels also identified numerous ongoing and serious challenges for PWA self-empowerment in the current phase of the epidemic. Looking forward, I highlight three trends emerging from the conference that have implications for the lives of people with HIV/AIDS and the PWA movement.

Stigma and Criminalization

In their special issue of the journal *Social Theory and Health* on HIV/AIDS in its third decade, Mykhalovskiy & Rosengarten (2009) call for critical social science research that examines "the growing global trend to criminalize HIV transmission/exposure" (p. 190). Indeed, it appears that issues of stigma and criminalization, once prevalent in the 1980s, have resurfaced as the disease has become — in the eyes of institutional authorities — normalized and treatable, in which case, by extension, transmission becomes an individual personal responsibility and punishable. In the most recently issue of POZ magazine the main story reads, "How Stigma Kills." The magazine did a poll of readers about the place of stigma in their lives and found, not surprisingly, that it pervaded many aspects of their lives. One comment from a reader read,

> Doctors won't accept me as a patient if I tell them up front that I'm HIV positive. Sometimes if I do get in with new doctors and they realize I'm HIV positive, they get mean or mad at me. People have made me wipe down everything I've used or touched with bleach. Living in a very rural redneck area of Florida, I take extra precautions to hide my status. Having gone to the local hospital ER [or to laboratories] for tests, I've had nurses drag other nurses or techs in to show me off like a sideshow at a circus. I see so much stigma here from the medical community it's appalling. Dental care is nonexistent for anyone HIV positive in my county due to stigma. (Hoffman, 2009)

Whereas education efforts have increased general knowledge and awareness about HIV/AIDS, there is evidence to suggest that attitudes toward people with the disease have not changed significantly in the last twenty-five years. Many people in the survey felt that the current anti-discrimination laws did not sufficiently serve their interests or protect their rights. At this moment in the epidemic, there are indications of greater institutional acceptance for people with HIV/AIDS. It is easier for people with HIV/AIDS to travel as countries change their border policies to accept those infected. Yet, the introduction of policies and legislation threatening to criminalize those infected for instances of transmission renews fears of recrimination, preventing people from disclosing and damaging efforts to reintegrate people with HIV/AIDS into social life. PWA organizations are renewing efforts to create safe places for people to disclose and be open about their health, both locally and globally, and advocating against criminal laws that persecute people with HIV/AIDS.

The Local and the Global

Delegates representing PWA organizations at the conference called for a global response to the ongoing challenges facing people with HIV/AIDS in impoverished social circumstances. This type of call to action is not distinct to this latest moment in the epidemic. People with HIV/AIDS have always demanded greater institutional involvement in fighting the disease. Moreover, since the early 1990s, if not earlier, PWA organizations recognized the need to frame the epidemic globally. What is distinct about this call to action is its emphasis on the local in addition to the global. With the intense globalization of the epidemic since 2000, people with HIV/AIDS and activists recognized that many people with HIV/AIDS in the developed world were also impoverished and increasingly becoming invisible. In his reflections on the conference in Mexico, Regan Hoffman (2008) writes

> As an American HIV-positive journalist, I blame, in part, the media for perpetuating the myth that AIDS is under control in America. It may be a crime of omission, but it is time that we give the rest of the world —as well as our current and future governmental leaders—a clear picture of what it's like to live with AIDS in America. If AIDS journalists in the United States aren't reporting on the key news about the American AIDS community, how will the rest of the world see that our own fight is far from over?

Hoffman's critique of the silence surrounding "AIDS in America" is another recurring theme emerging recently in PWA activism and organizing. This attention to the local is not necessarily a turn away from the needs and interests of people with HIV/AIDS in developing nations and around the world. Rather, the intent is to view a global response as one that recognizes self-empowerment and community development in the face of disadvantage, marginalization, and oppression as it occurs in developing and developed countries. An indication of this trend is in the November 2009 issue of *POZ* that highlights the power of local advocacy. In an editorial, Hoffman (2009) writes:

> The tipping point for AIDS advocacy has come. After more than a decade of denial about AIDS in America, a crisis of complacency within our government (with a handful of notable exceptions), infection rates that are higher than previously reported and levels of domestic funding for AIDS that are far from meeting the community's needs, it is time for all people living with and affected by HIV/AIDS to voice our concerns to those who will determine the health care of our futures.

The XVII International AIDS Conference brought the meetings back to North America and with that came a wider recognition that there was an insufficient institutional response to the epidemic in the United States and Canada. People with HIV/AIDS in developing countries are expressing similar concerns. Like the tone set in the *POZ* article — "Who Wants to be an AIDS Advocate" — the key to self-empowerment lies in fostering and building local capacity.

The Revival of GIPA

PWA organizing globally has increased significantly over the last decade. People with HIV/AIDS around the world are seeking to become more involved in the decisions that affect their lives. Accompanying this trend is a renewed commitment to the GIPA principle, one component of the PARIS declaration made at the Paris AIDS summit in 1994. The section of the declaration, signed by the Heads of Government or Representatives of 42 States, about the involvement of people with HIV/AIDS reads that we,

> support a greater involvement of people living with HIV/AIDS through an initiative to strengthen the capacity and coordination of networks of people living with HIV/AIDS and community-based organizations. By ensuring their full involvement in our common response to the pandemic at all - national, regional and global - levels, this initiative will, in particular, stimulate the creation of supportive political, legal and social environments. (Strub, 2008)

Even though the declaration is over fifteen years old, it is now a central document used to acknowledge the place of PWA organizing and activism in responding to the health crisis. In initiatives under UNAIDS the GIPA principle figured prominently. In 2008, for instance, UNAIDS released a policy brief that read, in part:

> People living with HIV understand each other's situation better than anyone and are often best placed to counsel one another and to represent their needs in decision- and policy-making forums. The idea that the personal experiences of people living with HIV could and should be translated into helping to shape a response to the AIDS epidemic was first voiced in 1983 at a national AIDS conference in the USA. It was formally adopted as a principle at the Paris AIDS Summit in 1994, where 42 countries declared the Greater Involvement of People Living with HIV and AIDS (GIPA) to be critical to ethical and effective national responses to the epidemic. Today the GIPA principle is the backbone of many interventions worldwide. People living with, or affected by HIV are involved in a wide variety of activities at all levels of the fight against AIDS; from appearing on posters, bearing personal testimony, and supporting and counselling others with HIV, to participating in major decision- and policy-making activities. (UNAIDS, 2008)

This endorsement of involvement brings the fight against HIV/AIDS by people with HIV/AIDS into a new institutional arena. It is a sign, on one level, that decision makers in government and international agencies are taking seriously PWA self-empowerment and community development. On another level, however, there is a concern that this acknowledgement is a step toward incorporating and muting activist efforts among people with HIV/AIDS to have their needs and interests addressed by institutional structures. In a cautionary tale about the threat of incorporation, Gregf Gonsalves (2005) writes about the problem of involving people with HIV/AIDS with a political commitment toward progressive social change:

> I am sick of GIPA and will not promote it any longer. It's time we start asking each other: What are you doing to promote the reproductive and sexual rights of women; to fight rape and violence against women; to promote access to HIV/AIDS prevention, care and treatment, to education, to safe and affordable housing and other basic services regardless of gender, sexuality, ethnic origin, regardless of ability to pay? What are you doing to legalize methadone, buprenorphine, syringe exchange and reform drug and narcotics regulation, protect sex workers from harassment, ensure they have working conditions that don't endanger their health or well-being? What are you doing to ensure that young people get comprehensive information about sexuality, STIs and HIV/AIDS? ... Let's base our personal commitment to the fight against HIV/AIDS not on who we are, but what we do for others and not just for those who are like us, but those who are different in whichever way each of us chooses to categorize it.

In this article, Gonsalves is not against the principle of greater involvement of people with HIV/AIDS per se, as much as he is calling for a renewed politics of engagement that recognizes the centrality of power, inequalities and oppression in the spread of HIV/AIDS. The revival of GIPA in international agencies and AIDS service organizations and PWA coalition organizations is a sign that PWA organizing and activism has acquired a legitimacy that has been illusive since the beginning of the epidemic. However, articulating a global response to the epidemic requires involving people with HIV/AIDS in a manner that is consistent with the "health from below" orientation that is central to the history of the PWA self empowerment movement.

The Importance of Counter Publics

International AIDS conferences feature prominently in this historical account of organizing and activism. Apart from the Second National AIDS Forum in Denver in 1983, which marked the beginning the PWA self-empowerment movement with the reading of the Denver Principles, each chapter has led with an account of one significant International AIDS Conference. In 1989 at the conference in Montreal, activists read the Montreal Manifesto, calling for greater institutional acceptance and involvement in the response to HIV/AIDS. At the Vancouver conference in 1996, scientists announced the benefits of HAART leading to the idea that the AIDS crisis was over. The conference in Durban, South Africa in 2000 marked the growing global awareness of the epidemic. Lastly, in Mexico in 2008 the EKAF declaration and the Mexico Manifesto may in time come to represent a new phrase in the epidemic in which the implications of non-infectiousness through treatment are apparent. Smith (2000) describes the meetings in this way:

> The International AIDS Conference might reasonably be called the "Olympics of AIDS." This biannual conference is, after all, the one event at which the best and brightest among the world's HIV/AIDS researchers, activists, and practitioners gather together, each time in a different, carefully selected city. And, like the Olympics, the event never fails to be steeped in politics or to generate media coverage...

A common theme across the conferences highlighted in this book is that people with HIV/AIDS have found a way to be actively involved in the proceedings. Early in the epidemic, people with HIV/AIDS were not welcomed at international scientific meetings. Only by taking over public proceedings and refusing to leave were they able to create space for people with HIV/AIDS at the International AIDS conference. The participation of people with HIV/AIDS in the conference is significant on many levels: a forum to express their needs and interests and to have expertise recognized; a meeting place and site for networking; and a contested terrain between activists, government officials and scientists. Since the

1990s, PWA organizations and networks have held their own conferences at times alongside scientific meetings or as an independent entity.

Creating forums for dialogue through the development of conferences, or creating a space in existing conferences, constitute a counter public sphere for people with HIV/AIDS. The formation of counter public spheres influences the transformative capacity of political activism and organizing (Fraser, 1992). As Marshall (1991) has argued, contemporary social movements - feminism, environmentalism, gay liberation - have each created counter public spheres through the development of social and cultural spaces. Social movement forums operate as counter publics on two levels. First, they provide a means for people to share and articulate their own expertise that can be used to critique existing forms of domination. Second, they provide a means for people to share their experiences and construct collective identities. It is in this way that social movements bring about social change: by creating a public sphere, they provide a means to articulate and put into practice alternative perspectives on ideas and meanings legitimated and reproduced through the dominant social order.

The history of publishing drawn upon in this study represents another means by which people with HIV/AIDS have contributed to the formation of a counter public sphere. It is possible to trace, over the course of the epidemic, an expansion and globalization of this counter pubic to the extent that is constitutes what Fraser refers to as a transnational public sphere (Bell, 2007). The rise of global networks of people with HIV/AIDS constitutes an important recent vehicle for dialogue and collaboration across political and geographic boundaries. Organizations, publications and conferences have been important in creating and sustaining a sense of solidarity among people with HIV/AIDS. In 1989, Slocum (1989) identified solidarity as an ongoing challenge for people with HIV/AIDS:

> It is very clear to me that our problems, those of living with this virus, are essentially the same all across the world. We are all inextricably intertwined in this "pandemic" but we have yet to find a global voice, or solidify an international network in which to share. Perhaps our work begins here at home. ... It is important that we work together to heal our brokenness at home. We need a united

voice. We need a united voice. We need our united strength. How else can we join in as partners in a global partnership to confront HIV? (p. 9)

Slocum's reflections are as relevant today as they were in 1989. In pointing out the need to find a global voice through building local capacity, he foreshadows many of the issues facing the PWA movement in 2009. Since the early 1980s people with HIV/AIDS have been, using the slogan of the movement, "Fighting for their Lives" by coming together collectively and insisting on being involved in the decisions that affect their survival. What is distinctive about PWA organizing and activism is that those involved realized early in the epidemic that the fight occurs on a symbolic level — a struggle over who determines what it means to be a person living with HIV/AIDS. Over the last twenty-five years, those involved in the PWA movement have responded to the changing landscape of the epidemic and struggled to change the institutionalized meanings generated about those living with HIV/AIDS. In the words of Sean Strub (2009) about the formation of the PWA movement in early 1980s during his remarks at the 2008 United States Conference on AIDS, "In the darkest days of the epidemic—when we were all frightened, when we were all suffering, when we were all angry—we knew what to do, and we did it."

References

A. (1997). Kids talk. *Women Alive Newsletter,* Retrieved January 17, 2009, from http://www.thebody.com/content/whatis/art167.html

ACT UP New York. (1996). AIDS profiteers declare war. Retrieved March 5, 2009, from http://www.actupny.org/Vancouver/declarewar.html

ACT UP New York. (2000). *Treatment for all... now!* Retrieved May 8, 2009 from http://www.actupny.org/reports/durban-access.html

Adam, B. (1987). *The rise of a gay and lesbian movement.* Boston: G.K. Hall Press.

Adam, B. & Sears, A. (1996). *Experiencing HIV.* New York: Columbia University Press.

AIDS ACTION NOW! & ACT UP New York. (1989). *Le manifeste de Montreal.* Retrieved May 8, 2009 from http://www.gaylib.com/text/misc12.htm

AIDS at 25: Looking back moving forward. (2006, June). *Outreach, 4*(20), 1.

Altman, D. (1982). *The homosexualization of America.* Boston: Beacon Press.

Altman, D. (1986). *AIDS in the mind of America.* Garden City, N.Y.: Doubleday Press.

Altman, D. (1994). *Power and community: Organizational and cultural responses to AIDS.* Social aspects of AIDS. London: Taylor & Francis.

Altman, D. (1999). Globalization, political economy, and HIV/AIDS. *Theory and Society. 28*(4), 559-584.

Altman, L. K. (1991, June 18). W.H.O. says 40 million will be infected with AIDS virus by 2000. *New York Times.* Retrieved May 4, 2009, from http://www.nytimes.com/library/national/science/aids/061891sci-aids.html

American Association for World Health. (2001, December 1). Why we should care: 20 years of AIDS — 1981 to 2001. *I care...do you? Youth and AIDS in the 21st Century.* Retrieved June 8, 2009, from http://www.thebody.com/content/art33030.html

Anderson, W. (1994, July). News and notes: In the courts — two wins. *Body Positive*, p. 9.

Andriote, J. M. (1999). *Victory deferred: How AIDS changed gay life in America.* Chicago: University of Chicago Press.

Ariss, R. (1996). *Against death: The practice of living with AIDS.* Australia: Gordon & Breach Publishers.

Ariss, R. M., & Dowsett, G. W. (1997). *Against death: The practice of living with AIDS.* Theory and practice in medical anthropology and international health, v. 5. Australia: Gordon and Breach.

Armstrong, W. (1999, December). The AIDS decade: The 99 greatest moments of the '90s. *POZ Magazine.* Retrieved March 3, 2009, from http://www.poz.com/articles/221_1547.shtml

Baker, M. (2002, January/February). Mobilizing the troops: Newly international North American activist alliance gathers in Vancouver. *Tagline.* Retrieved February 17, 2009, from http://www.thebody.com/content/art1667.html

Barr, D. (2003, April). Tipping point: MSF, Oxfam redefine the possible, and Y2K activist trek to Durban marks a watershed. *Tagline.* Retrieved May 11, 2009 from http://www.thebody.com/content/art1767.html

Barr, D. (2003, March). Yin and Yang. *Tagline.* Retrieved March 2, 2009, from http://www.thebody.com/content/confs/art1595.html

Barr, M. (1994, June/July). Essay: world AIDS conference. *POZ Magazine, 2.* Retrieved May 12, 2009 from http://www.poz.com/articles/262_15858.shtml

Barr, M. (1997, February). The morning after. *POZ Magazine.* Retrieved March 18, 2009, from http://www.poz.com/articles/237_1691.shtml

Barr, M. (2003, March). Yokohama, Vancouver, twin Pacific ports, serve as polar opposites for scientific advances. *TAGline.* Retrieved March 20, 2009, from http://www.thebody.com/content/art1595.html

Bayer R. (1986). AIDS, power, and reason. *The Milbank Quarterly.* 64, 168-82.

Bayer, R. (1991). Covering the plague: AIDS and the American media. *AIDS Education and Prevention*, 3(1), 74-86.

Bell, V. (2007). The Potential of an "Unfolding Constellation": Imagining Fraser's transnational public sphere. *Theory, Culture & Society,* 24(4), 1-5.

Bernard, E. (2008). Swiss experts say individuals with undetectable viral load and no STI cannot transmit HIV during sex. *AIDSmap.* Retrieved December 10, 2009, from http://www.aidsmap.com/en/news/4E9D555B-18FB-4D56-B912-2C28AFCCD36B.asp

Body Positive. (2006). 25 Years of AIDS: A Timeline. *Body Positive Magazine* (2). Retrieved December 5, 2009, from http://www.thebody.com/content/art31152.html

Bordowitz, G. (2001, May). What the world needs now. *POZ Magazine*, 70. Retrieved May 13, 2009 from http://www.poz.com/articles/188_1157.shtml

Bornhoeft, M.-A. (1998, January). News & notes. *Body Positive*. Retrieved May 8, 2009 from http://www.thebody.com/content/art30966.html

Brouwer, D. (2005). Counterpublicity and corporeality in HIV/AIDS zines. *Critical Studies in Media Communication*. (22)5, December, 351-371.

Brown, M. P. (1997). *Replacing citizenship: AIDS activism and radical democracy*. Mappings. New York: Guilford Press.

C. (1992, September). Positive women. *Living Positive*, (59), 4.

C. L. (1988, January). The shiny black bowl. *Body Positive*, *1*(2), 9.

Cadman, J & Kaminski, D. (2000, September/October). Success in preventing mother-to-child transmission not a reality for all. *GMHC Treatment Issues*. Retrieved May 26, 2009 from http://www.thebody.com/content/art13216.html

Cain, R. (1993). *AIDS service organizations in context: An interim report*. Hamilton: School of Social Work, McMaster University.

Cain, R. (1993). Community-based AIDS services: Formalization and depoliticization. *International Journal of Health Services: Planning, Administration, Evaluation, 23*(4), 665-84.

Califia-Rice, P. (2001, January). Magical mystery cure. *POZ Magazine*. Retrieved March 17, 2009, from http://www.poz.com/articles/185_1038.shtml

Callen, M. & Turner, D. (1997, December). A history of the People With AIDS self-empowerment movement. *Body Positive*. Retrieved April 4, 2008, from http://www.thebody.com/content/art31074.html

Callen, M. (1985, November). The body politic. *PWA Coalition Newsline*, (5), 10.

Callen, M. (1987). Introduction. In M. Callen's (Ed) *Surviving and thriving with AIDS: Hints for the newly diagnosed* (p. ix). New York: People with AIDS Coalition.

Callen, M. (1987). *Surviving and thriving with AIDS: Hints for the newly diagnosed*. New York: People with AIDS Coalition.

Callen, M. (1987). Treating opportunistic infections and AIDS itself. In M. Callen's (Ed). *Surviving and thriving with AIDS: Hints for the newly diagnosed* (35-42). New York: People with AIDS Coalition.

Callen, M. (1990). *Surviving AIDS*. New York, NY: HarperCollins.

Carbone, D. (1996, November). Under lock and key: Living with HIV/AIDS in youth lock-ups. *Body Positive*, p. 14.

Carter, E. & Watney, S. (1989). *Taking liberties: AIDS and cultural politics*. London: Serpent's Tail in association with the ICA.

Carter, G. (2002, April). Fighting back against pharmaceutical company greed. *GMHC Treatment Issues*. Retrieved March 30, 2009, from http://www.thebody.com/content/policy/art13653.html

Cassidy, W. P. (2005). Accent on the POZ? AIDS coverage in POZ, a magazine for HIV-positive individuals. *Atlantic Journal of Communication, 13*(3), 169-182.

Chambré, S. M. (2006). *Fighting for our lives: New York's AIDS community and the politics of disease*. Critical issues in health and medicine. New Brunswick, N.J.: Rutgers University Press.

Clarke, J. (1993). *Burlington breast cancer support services*. Waterloo: Wilfrid Laurier University: Unpublished Manuscript.

Cochrane, M. (2004). *When AIDS began: San Francisco and the making of an epidemic*. New York: Routledge.

Counter, M. (1996). A history of the people living with HIV/AIDS (PLWHA) movement in Australia. *Social Alternatives, 15*(4), 25-27.

Courson, F. L. (1999, September/October). Time-out/time-in suspending one's drug regimen. *Positively Aware*. Retrieved March 26, 2009, from http://www.thebody.com/content/art883.html

Coyle, H. (1996, November). Uncommon Curtis. *POZ Magazine*, (18), 40.

Crawford. R. (1994). The boundaries of the self and the unhealthy other: Reflections on health, culture, and AIDS. *Social Science & Medicine, 38*(10), 1347-1365.

Crimp, D. (1988). *AIDS: cultural analysis, cultural activism*. Cambridge, Mass: MIT Press.

Crimp, D. (1990). *AIDS demographics*. Seattle: Bay Press.

Crimp, D. (2004). *Melancholia and moralism: Essays on AIDS and queer politics*. Cambridge, Mass: MIT.

Cullinan, K. & Thom, A. (2000, July). An international incident. *POZ Magazine*, 61. Retrieved May 27, 2009 from http://www.poz.com/articles/203_10298.shtml

Currier, J. (1994, September). Henry for president. *Body Positive*, p. 10.

Currier, J. (1994, August). Hugh Steers: Portrait of an artist in the epidemic. *Body Positive*, 16-19.

d'Adesky, A. (2007, July 11). Never say never in Nairobi: Africa hosts a women's summit on HIV. *POZ Magazine*. Retrieved May 19, 2009 from http://www.poz.com/articles/women_hiv_nairobi_401_12534.shtml

Daniel, D. (1994, October/November). Swing shift. *POZ Magazine, 1*(4), 20.

De Moor, K. (2005). Diseased pariahs and difficult patients. *Cultural Studies, 19*(6), 737-754.

DeGagne, D. (1989, September/October). Montreal Fifth International Conference on AIDS. *Vancouver PWA Coalition Newsletter*, (31), 4.

Delaney, M. (1999, December). Happy holidays? *POZ Magazine*, (54). Retrieved March 24, 2009, from http://www.poz.com/articles/221_1549.shtml

Delaney, M. (2001, July). It's raining meds. *POZ Magazine*, (72). Retrieved March 26, 2009, from http://www.poz.com/articles/190_1213.shtml

Delaney, M. (2002, April). Opinion: The looming crisis in drug pricing. *GMHC Treatment Issues*. Retrieved March 30, 2009, from http://www.thebody.com/content/policy/art13652.html

Dowd, M. (1994, October/November). Proud Mary. *POZ Magazine, 1*(4), 32.

Drake, D. (1999, May). When plagues return. *POZ Magazine*, p. 20.

Dreifus, C. (1970). *Seizing our bodies: The politics of the women's health movement*. New York: Vintage.

Dugdale, J. (1995, June/July). His mind's eye. *POZ Magazine*, (8), 55-56.

Duttman, A. (1996). *At odds with AIDS: Thinking and talking about a virus.* Standford: Stanford University Press.

Editor. (2000, April). POZ Alternatives. *POZ Magazine*, p. 45.

Editors. (1999, July). The power of one. *POZ Magazine*, 49. Retrieved May 13, 2009 from http://www.poz.com/articles/216_1530.shtml

Elliot, A. (2003, Winter). Depression and HIV in the era of HAART. *STEP Perspective*. Retrieved December 5, 2009, from http://www.thebody.com/content/art1819.html

Epstein, S. (1991). Democratic science? AIDS activism and the contested construction of knowledge. *Socialist Review, 21*(2) 35-64.

Epstein S. (1995). The construction of lay expertise: AIDS activism and the forging of credibility in the reform of clinical *trials. Science, Technology & Human Values.* 20(4), 408-37.

Epstein S. (1996). Impure science: AIDS, activism, and the politics of knowledge. *Medicine and Society.* 1-466.

F., J. (1988, October). Loaded dice. *Body Positive, 1*(10), 11.

Fee, E., & Fox, D. M. (1988). *AIDS: The burdens of history.* Berkeley: University of California Press.

Fee, E., & Fox, D.M. (1992). *AIDS: The making of a chronic disease.* Berkley: University of California Press.

Feuer, C. (2002, October). Worlds collide. *POZ Magazine*, 85. Retrieved May 26, 2009 from http://www.poz.com/articles/181_972.shtml

Flowers, P. (2001). Gay men and HIV/AIDS risk management. *Health.* 5 (1), 50-75.

Fox, D.M. (1992) The politics of HIV infection: 1989-1990 as years of change. In E. Fee & D.M. Fox (Eds.), *AIDS: The making of a chronic disease.* Berkley: University of California Press.

Fraser, N. (1992). "Rethinking the public sphere: A contribution to the critique of actually existing democracy." In C. Calhoun (Ed.), *Habermas and the Public Sphere.* (pp. 109-142). Cambridge: MIT Press.

Freidson, E. (2007). Professional dominance: The social structure of medical care. New Brunswick, NJ: Aldine Transaction.

Gamson, J. (1989). Silence, death, and the invisible enemy: AIDS activism and social movement newness. *Social Problems, 36*(4), 351-367.

Geffen, N. (2000, September/October). What happened in Durban? A South African perspective. *Treatment Issues.* Retrieved May 27, 2009 from http://www.thebody.com/content/art13213.html

Gendin, S. (2000, April). On the runs. *POZ Magazine,* p. 41.

Gilden, D. (2000, April). Adverse events. *POZ Magazine,* p. 40.

Gilman, S. L., (1988). *Disease and representation: Images of illness from madness to AIDS.* Cornell University Press, Ithaca, NY.

Goldberg, R. (1998, July). Conference call: When PWAs first sat at the high table. *POZ Magazine,* (37). Retrieved July 28, 2008, from http://www.poz.com/articles/229_7188.shtml

Goldstein, R. (1998, October). Climb every mountain. *POZ Magazine,* (40). Retrieved March 27, 2009 from http://www.poz.com/articles/232_12193.shtml

Gonsalves, G. (2005). Rage against the machine. Anti-politics and the AIDS epidemic. GMHC Treatment Issues, Retrieved December 10, 2009 from http://www.thebody.com/content/art13606.html

Gore, J. (2002). What we can do for you! What can "we" do for "you"?: Struggling over empowerment in critical and feminist pedagogy. In A. Darder, M. Baltodano & R. D. Torres (Eds.), *The Critical Pedagogy Reader* (pp. 331-348). New York: Routledge.

Graham, J. (2006, January/February). 25 years of AIDS and HIV: A look back 1981-1986: In the Beginning. *Survival News.* Retrieved June 11, 2009, from http://www.thebody.com/content/whatis/art32414.html

Greenwood, J. (1999, April). Going on holiday. *Survival News.* Retrieved March 24, 2009, from http://www.thebody.com/content/treat/art32510.html

Greenwood, J. (2000, December). Burned out? Join the club! Survival News. Retrieved March 24, 2009, from http://www.thebody.com/content/art32473.html

Grinberg, L. (1999, May). Honeymoon to HAARTache. *POZ Magazine*, (47). Retrieved March 24, 2009, from http://www.poz.com/articles/ 214_1526.shtml

Hale, J. (1989). After Montreal, international AIDS conferences will never be the same. *Canadian Medical Association Journal, 141*(2), 144-146.

Harrington, M. (2000, December). Brazil: what went right? *Tagline.* Retrieved May 19, 2009 from http://www.thebody.com/content/policy/art1723.html

Harrington, M. (2006, December). Editorial: what's next? *Tagline.* Retrieved May 13, 2009 from http://www.thebody.com/content/policy/art39863.html

Harris, P. (1994, June). Sports for all...that means you. *Body Positive*, p. 13.

Harris, P. (1995, August). Stepping out. *Body Positive*, p. 12.

Hattoy, B. (1998, October). Table of contents. *POZ Magazine*, p. 8.

Hemp, M. (2004, Winter). Interview with Lillian Mworeko. *Positives for Positives*, 28. Retrieved May 19, 2009 from http://img.thebody.com/ legacyAssets/49/22/winter04.pdf

Herdt, G. H., & Lindenbaum, S. (1992). *The time of AIDS: Social analysis, theory, and method.* Newbury Park: Sage Publications.

Highleyman, L. (2004, January 30). What were the Denver Principles? *Gmax.co.za*, Retrieved April 10, 2008, from http://www.gmax.co.za/ think/history/2004/040130-bobbicampbell.html

HIV abroad (1989, June). *Body Positive, 2*(5), 21.

"HIV Man" (1987). More thoughts about AL 721. In M. Callen (Ed.), *Surviving and thriving with AIDS: Hints for the newly diagnosed* (p. 54). New York: People with AIDS Coalition.

Hofmann, R. (2008). Fight Club: Reflections on Mexico City. POZ Magazine, Retreived December 10, 2009 from http://www.poz.com/articles/ iac_reflections_aids_401_15219.shtml

Hofmann, R. (2009). How stigma kills. *POZ Magazine*, Retrieved December 10, 2009 from http://www.poz.com/articles/how_stigma_kills_hiv_2416 _17574.shtml

Hofmann, R. (2009). Who wants to be an AIDS advocate? *POZ Magazine.* Retrieved December 10, 2009 from http://www.poz.com/articles/hiv_ advocacy_hub_november_2397_17440.shtml

Holtgrave D. R. (2005). Causes of the decline in AIDS deaths, United States, 1995-2002: Prevention, treatment or both? *International Journal of STD & AIDS* 16, 777-781.

Horowitz, R. (1997, February). Kvitch: 1987: silence=death 1997: apathy=more death. *Body Positive.* Retrieved March 30, 2009, from http://www.thebody.com/content/art31023.html

Horowitz, R. (1997, June). Under two hundred: all the invisible lines in the world of AIDS. *Body Positive*. Retrieved June 11, 2009, from http://www.thebody.com/content/art30771.html

Illiffe, J. (2007). *The African AIDS epidemic: A history*. Athens: Ohio University Press.

In our new office at last. (1986, October). *Vancouver PWA Coalition Newsletter*, (1), 1.

International Community of Women Living with HIV/AIDS. (2006). *ICW introduction and history*. Retrieved May 15, 2009 from http://www.icw.org/about-ICW

James, D. (1990, January). Living with hemophilia. *Body Positive*, *3*(1), 12.

James, J. S. (1996, June). "Access for all": Communication strategy proposal for activists at International Conference. *AIDS Treatment News*. Retrieved March 5, 2009, from http://www.thebody.com/content/art31482.html#Access

James, J. S. (1997, January). Aids treatment news January 17th, 1997. *AIDS Treatment News*, Retrieved March 5, 2009, from http://www.thebody.com/content/art31497.html

James, J. S. (1999, April 16). New frontier of AIDS activism. *AIDS Treatment News*. Retrieved May 20, 2009 from http://www.thebody.com/content/art31551.html#global_access

James, J. S. (1999, November 1). Pharmaceutical patents and developing countries. *AIDS Treatment News*. Retrieved May 19, 2009 from http://www.thebody.com/content/art31564.html#patents

James, J. S. (2000, September 22). Brazil AIDS success: Washington Post report. *AIDS Treatment News*. Retrieved May 8, 2009 from http://www.thebody.com/content/world/art32060.html

James, J. S. (2000, December 1). Global treatment access: call for 95% price reduction. *AIDS Treatment News*. Retrieved May 20, 2009 from http://www.thebody.com/content/art32030.html

James, J. S. (2001, December 28). AIDS treatment news denialist series. *AIDS Treatment News*. Retrieved May 28, 2009 from http://www.thebody.com/content/art31889.html

James, J. S. (2001, July 27). Global Epidemic, U.S. Response: a winning strategy, what you can do. *AIDS Treatment News*. Retrieved May 11, 2009 from http://www.thebody.com/content/art31939.html

James, J. S. (2003, September 12). Nevirapine reduced mother-to-child transmission better than AZT — at 70 times less cost. *AIDS Treatment News*. Retrieved May 26, 2009 from http://www.thebody.com/content/art31749.html

Joint United Nations Programme on HIV/AIDS. (2004). *Report on the global AIDS epidemic, 2004.* [Geneva]: Joint United Nations Programme on HIV/AIDS.

Kahn, A. D. (1993). *AIDS, the winter war.* Philadelphia: Temple University Press.

Kaplan, L. (1995, April/May). My brother, my self. *POZ Magazine,* (7), 34.

Keeley, C. (1995, August/September). Women on the verge. *POZ Magazine,* (9), 50.

King, C. (2007, February 23). Charles King's speech on "The future of the AIDS movement -lessons from New Orleans." *POZ Magazine.* Retrieved May 28, 2009 from http://www.poz.com/articles/401_11380.shtml

King, M. S. (1999, May). Lazarus gets a third wind. *Body Positive.* Retrieved March 12, 2009, from http://www.thebody.com/content/art30643.html

Kinsman, G. (1987). *The regulation of desire: sexuality in Canada.* Montreal: Black Rose Press.

Kinsman, G. (1991). "Their silence, our deaths": What can the social sciences offer to AIDS research? In D. Goldstein (Ed.), Talking AIDS: Interdisciplinary perspectives on *AIDS (pp.* 39-60). St. John's, NF: Institute for Social and Economic Research (ISER) Policy Papers.

Kirp, D. L. & Bayer, R. (1992). *AIDS in the industrialized democracies: Passions, politics, and policies.* New Brunswick, N.J.: Rutgers University Press.

Knight, L. (2008). *UNAIDS the first ten years, 1996-2006.* Geneva, Switzerland: Joint United Nations Programme on HIV/AIDS (UNAIDS).

Kramer, L. (2007, March 14). We are not crumbs; we must not accept crumbs. *POZ Magazine,* Retrieved June 11, 2009, from http://www.poz.com/articles/401_11492.shtml

Kurth, P. (1997, December). Once upon a Lazarus. *POZ Magazine.* Retrieved March 13, 2009, from http://www.poz.com/articles/resurrection_bible_ aids_246_12858.shtml

Lands, L. (1998, September). The circle game. *POZ Magazine,* (39). Retrieved March 29, 2009, from http://www.poz.com/articles/231_7412.shtml

Lands, L. (2000, September). Pills! Chills! Thrills! Spills! *POZ Magazine,* (63). Retrieved December 5, 2009, from http://www.poz.com/articles/ 205_10153.shtml

Lederer, B. & Brownworth, V. A. (1997, April). The price may not be right. *POZ Magazine,* (22). Retrieved March 30, 2009, from http://www.poz.com/ articles/239_1710.shtml

Leonardis, O. & Mauri, D. (1992). From deinstitutionalization to the social enterprise. *Social Policy, 25*(3), 50-54.

Levy, D. (1998, January). To be young, black, and a one-man AIDS epidemic. *Body Positive*. Retrieved January 16, 2009 from http://www.thebody.com/content/art30963.html

Lewis, J. (1990, November). Out of the HIV closet. *Body Positive, 3*(9), 19.

LHIVE, (2008). The Mexico Manifesto. *LHIVE*. Retrieved December 10, 2009 from http://www.lhive.ch/73901/index.html

Licata, S. (1987, July/August). Protesting at the International AIDS Conference. *PWA Coalition Newsline,* (25), 2.

Link, D. (2000, September/October). Reading Durban. *Treatment Issues*. Retrieved May 11, 2009 from http://www.thebody.com/content/art13215.html

Long, T. L. (2000). Plague of pariahs: AIDS' zines and the rhetoric of transgression. *Journal of Communication Inquiry*, 24, 401-411.

Lubow, A. (1995, May 1). Talk of the town: Positive thinking. *New Yorker*, p. 32.

Lupton, D. (1994). *Moral threats and dangerous desires: AIDS in the news media*. Social aspects of AIDS. London: Taylor & Francis.

Lupton, D. (1999). Archetypes of infection: People with HIV/AIDS in the Australian press in the mid 1990s. *Sociology of Health and Illness 21,*(1), 37-53.

MacInnis, R. (2006). The International AIDS Conference: A retrospective—do we need more? *Global AIDSLink, 8*, 14.

MacLachlan, J. (1992). Managing AIDS: A phenomenology of experiment, empowerment and expediency, *Critique of Anthropology*. (12) 4, Dec, 433-456.

Maldonado, M. (1999, February). State of emergency: HIV/AIDS among African Americans. *Body Positive*. Retrieved January 16, 2009, from http://www.thebody.com/content/art31002.html

Mallet, M. (1988, November). AIDS hysteria in San Francisco. *PWA Coalition Newsline, 38*, 56.

Mann, J. M. & Tarantola, D. (1996). *AIDS in the world II: Global dimensions, social roots, and responses*. New York: Oxford University Press.

Mars, A. (1994, January). Tom Duane. *Body Positive*, p. 16.

Marsh, M. (1995, September). Moment of truth: A teenager's story. *Body Positive*, p. 10.

Marshall, B. (1991). "Communication as politics: Feminist print media in English Canada." *Women's Studies International Forum*. (18)4, 463-474.

Martin, M. (1997, March). Monkey business — Jeff Getty talks about life after baboons. *POZ Magazine,* (21), 111.

Martin, M. (1997, September). Checking in. *POZ Magazine,* (27). Retrieved March 29, 2009, from http://www.poz.com/articles/244_13609.shtml

Maxwell, C., Aggleton, P., Warwick, I. (2008). Involving HIV-positive people in policy and service development: recent experiences in England. *AIDS Care,* 20(1), 72-79.

Menadue, D. (2008, September). Criminal laws condemned at Mexico. *POSLINK: The Newsletter of People Living with HIV/AIDS Victoria,* (41), 1-7.

McCabe, L. (1997, Summer). Intolerant, resistant but still complying. *Women Alive Newsletter.* Retrieved March 20, 2009, from http://www.thebody.com/content/treat/art163.html

Milano, M. (2001, January/February). 2000: A year of endings and beginnings. *Positively Aware.* Retrieved May 18, 2009 from http://www.thebody.com/content/art1259.html

Miller, J. (1992). *Fluid exchanges: Artists and critics in the AIDS crisis.* Toronto: University of Toronto Press.

Miller, K. (1996, December). Starving to death to live: Crixivan — the newest "silver bullet" in AIDS treatment! *Body Positive.* Retrieved March 27, 2009, from http://www.thebody.com/content/living/art31083.html

Minnich, B. (1996, November). Citizen Duane. *POZ Magazine,* (18), 38.

Minnich, B. (1999, October). Northern Light. *POZ Magazine,* (52), p. 87.

Mirken, B. (2000, December 1). Answering the AIDS denialists: Is AIDS real? *AIDS Treatment News.* Retrieved May 27, 2009 from http://www.thebody.com/content/art32028.html

Moore, G. (1993, January). SAGE: Addressing seniors with AIDS. *Body Positive,* 6(1), 7.

Morris, D. (2001, November/December). Living with HIV. *Positively Aware.* Retrieved March 24, 2009, from http://www.thebody.com/content/treat/art1001.html

Morris, K. (1994, July). Women prisoners with HIV speak out: At Muncy, PA. *Women Alive Newsletter.* Retrieved January 17, 2009, from http://www.thebody.com/content/whatis/art225.html

Morris, S. (1997, June). Re-evaluating the miracle cocktail. *Body Positive.* Retrieved March 18, 2009, from http://www.thebody.com/content/art30769.html

Morrison, M. (1991, October). Positively pregnant. *Body Positive,* 4(8), 14.

Mykhalovskiy, E., Mccoy, L., & Bresalier, M. (2004). Compliance/adherence, HIV, and the critique of medical power. *Social Theory & Health* 2(4), 315-340.

Mykhalovskiy, E. & Rosengarten, M. (2009). HIV/AIDS in its third decade: Renewed critique in social and cultural analysis — An introduction. *Social Theory & Health* (7), 187-195.

Natale, R. (1995, December/January). Hollywood shuffles AIDS. *POZ Magazine*, (11), 58.

Navarre, M. (1985, November). A queen screams. *PWA Coalition Newsline*, (6), 11-12.

Navarre, M. (1985, September). Go west young man. *PWA Coalition Newsline*, (4), 9.

Navarre, M. (1988). Fighting the victim label. In D. Crimp (Ed.), *AIDS: cultural analysis/cultural activism* (pp. 143-146). Cambridge, MA: MIT Press.

Navarre, M. (1988). PWA coalition portfolio. In D. Crimp (Ed.), *AIDS: cultural analysis/cultural activism* (pp. 147-168). Cambridge, MA: MIT Press.

Nine, G. (1988, November). The cure is happening now. *PWA Coalition Newsline, 38*, 34.

Palmer, J. (2004, Fall). Final thoughts after Bangkok: Women, HIV and gender-based violence. *Positive for Positives*. Retrieved May 28, 2009 from http://www.thebody.com/content/art4941.html

Patton, C. (1985). *Sex and germs: The politics of AIDS*. Boston: South End Press.

Patton, C. (1990). *Inventing AIDS*. New York: Routledge.

Patton, C. (1994). *Last served?: Gendering the HIV pandemic*. Bristol, PA: Taylor and Francis.

Pawluch, D., Cain, R., & Gillett, J. (1994). Ideology and alternative therapy use among people living with HIV/AIDS. *Health and Canadian Society, 2*(1), 63-84.

Pawluch, D., Cain, R., & Gillett, J. (2000). Lay constructions of HIV and complementary therapy use. *Social Science and Medicine* 51: 251-264.

Perez, J. C. (1996, June/July). The heat is on. *POZ Magazine*, (15), 35.

Persson, A. (2004). Incorporating pharmakon: HIV, medicine, and body shape change. *Body & Society* 10, 45-67.

Persson, A., Race, K., & Wakeford, E. (2003). HIV health in context: Negotiating medical technology and lived experience. *Health: An Interdisciplinary Journal for the Social Study of Health, Illness and Medicine* 7, 397-415.

Pickett, J. (1999, September/October). I'm dancing as fast as I can. *Positively Aware*. Retrieved March 24, 2009, from http://www.thebody.com/content/art882.html

Pickett, J. (2000, May/June). Stop the drugs — a personal détente. *Positively Aware*. Retrieved March 30, 2009, from http://www.thebody.com/content/art1077.html

Pickett, J. (2002, September/October). Test positive aware network turns 15. *Positively Aware*, 52-53. Retrieved January 16, 2009, from http://www.thebody.com/content/art925.html

Poku, N. (2002). Global pandemics: HIV/AIDS. In D. Held & A. G. McGrew (Eds.), *Governing globalization: Power, authority, and global governance* (pp.111-126). Cambridge: Polity.

Positive Youth Outreach. (n.d.) *About us.* Retrieved January 17, 2009, from http://www.positiveyouth.com/static/aboutus.html

Prescott, L. (1996, October). Medical highlights from the Eleventh International Conference on AIDS. *Body Positive.*

Project Inform. (2000, August). Denial defeated, hope reigns. *Perspective.* Retrieved May 7, 2009, from http://www.thebody.com/content/whatis/art5827.html

Project Inform. (2000, October). Durban: between the lines. *Perspective.* Retrieved May 7, 2009, from http://www.thebody.com/content/art5509.html

Project Inform. (2000, October). Women at Durban. *Perspective.* Retrieved May 25, 2009, from http://www.thebody.com/content/world/art5513.html

Project Inform. (2003, January). The challenge of Barcelona. *Perspective.* Retrieved May 26, 2009, from http://www.thebody.com/content/policy/art5600.html

R. (1992, July/August). Prison notes. *Living Positive*, (8), 19.

R. (1992, July/August). Women and HIV. *Living Positive*, (58), 26.

Randolph, L. B. (1997, April) Exclusive! Cookie Johnson on: the Magic "miracle." "The Lord has healed Earvin." *Ebony, 52.*

Rayside, D. & Lindquist, E. (1992). Canada: Community activism, federalism and the new politics of disease. In D. Kirp & R. Bayer (Eds.) *AIDS in the industrialized democracies: Passions, politics and policies* (pp. 49-98). New Brunswick, N.J.: Rutgers University Press, and Montreal: McGill-Queen's Univ. Press.

Roberts Auli, C. (1995, Summer). A global community: PWA conference. *Women Alive.* Retrieved May 14, 2009 from http://www.thebody.com/content/art204.html

Rodriguez, E. (1999, December/ 2000, January). Safety concerns prompt suspension of Lodenosine clinical trial. *Positive Living.* Retrieved March 28, 2009, from http://www.thebody.com/content/treat/art32794.html

Rofes, E. E. (1998). *Dry bones breathe: Gay men creating post-AIDS identities and cultures.* Haworth gay & lesbian studies. New York: Haworth Press.

Rolands, P. (1997, Spring). My adventures with Crixivan or toxic side effects, anyone? *Women Alive Newsletter.* Retrieved March 27, 2009, from http://www.thebody.com/content/treat/art332.html

Rosenbrock, R., Dubois-Arber, F., Moers, M., Pinell, P., Schaeffer, D., & Setbon, M. (2000). The normalization of AIDS in Western European countries. *Social Science & Medicine. 50*(11), 1607-29.

Rosett, J. (1997, March). The buddy line. *POZ Magazine*. (21). Retrieved June 2, 2008, from http://www.poz.com/articles/238_12500.shtml

Roy, C. (1995). *Living and serving: Persons with HIV in the Canadian AIDS movement*. Ottawa, ON: Canadian AIDS Society.

Roy, C. & Cain, R. (2001). The involvement of people living with HIV/AIDS in community-based organizations: Contributions and constraints. *AIDS CARE 13*(4), 421-432.

Sacks, R. (1999, December). Issues in integrative medicine: Complementary and alternative medicine conference: Part 1. *Body Positive*. Retrieved March 29, 2009, from http://www.thebody.com/content/art31057.html

Salyer, D. (2000, September). Queens of denial. *Survival News*. Retrieved May 27, 2009 from http://www.thebody.com/content/whatis/art32220.html

Salyer, D. (2006, June/July). Cruising with Lazarus. *Survival News*. Retrieved June 10, 2009, from http://www.thebody.com/content/art32372.html

San Francisco AIDS Foundation. *I am Worth*. Retrieved November 17, 2009, from http://www.sfaf.org/aboutsfaf/gallery/worth.cfm

Santee, B. (1988). HIV positive women have rights too and they're often denied. *On The Issues,* 10. Retrieved January 16, 2009, from http://www.ontheissuesmagazine.com/1988vol10/vol10_1988_2.php

Savage, T. (1996, January). People's choice. *POZ Magazine*, (18), 38.

Sawyer, E. (1996, July). Remarks at the opening ceremony. *ACT UP New York*. Retrieved March 5, 2009, from http://www.actupny.org/Vancouver/sawyerspeech.html

Schick, R. (1988, November). A good attitude is nice, but it won't cure AIDS. *PWA Coalition Newsline*, (38), 50.

Schoofs, M. (1995, April/May). Time after Times. *POZ Magazine*, (7), 28.

Sears, A. (1991). AIDS and the health of nations: The contradictions of public health. *Critical Sociology 18*(2), 31-50.

Seckinelgin, H. (2003). HIV/AIDS, global civil society and people's politics. In: M. Kaldor, H. Anheier, & M. Glasius (Eds.), *Global civil society 2003* (pp.422-424). Oxford: Oxford University Press.

Segal, L. (1989). Lessons from the past: Feminism, sexual politics and the challenge of AIDS, in E. Carter & S. Watney (Eds.) *Taking liberties: AIDS and cultural politics*. London: Serpent's Tail in association with the ICA.

Selwyn, P. A., & Arnold, R. (1998, December) From fate to tragedy: The changing meanings of life, death, and AIDS. *Annals of Internal Medicine 129*(11), Pt. 1, 899-902.

Shernoff, M. (1997, March). Challenges and dilemmas regarding protease inhibitors. *Body Positive*, p. 15.

Shernoff, M. & Smith, R. A. (2000, November). To med or not to med? *Body Positive.* Retrieved March 26, 2009, from http://www.thebody.com/content/treat/art30639.html

Silversides, A. (2003). *AIDS activist Michael Lynch and the politics of community.* Toronto [Ont.]: Between the Lines.

Sky. (1987). Dear brother and sisters. In M. Callen (Ed) *Surviving and thriving with AIDS: Collected wisdom* (p. 264). New York: People with AIDS Coalition.

Slocum, M. (1989, November). Fighting HIV in communities of colour. *Body Positive, 2*(8), 12.

Slocum, M. (1989, July/August). In search of community. *Body Positive, 2*(6), 7-9.

Slocum, M. (1989, July/August). Science meets activism. *Body Positive, 2*(6), 8-13.

Slocum, M. (1990, February). From the editor. *Body Positive, 3*(1), 9.

Slocum, M. & Lewis, J. (19982, December 31, Revised January 12, 2009). You are not alone. *Body Positive.* Retrieved May 8, 2008, from http://www.thebody.com/content/art30259.html

Smith, G. (1990). Political activist as ethnographer. *Social Problems, 37*(4), 629-648.

Smith, R. A. (2000, October). The Durban Declaration. *Body Positive.* Retrieved May 8, 2009, from http://www.thebody.com/content/whatis/art30547.html

Smith, R. A. (2001, August). Global AIDS: The big picture. *Body Positive.* Retrieved May 13, 2009 from http://www.thebody.com/content/policy/art31196.html

Smith, R. A. (2001, January). Two decades of AIDS: Scenes from an epidemic. *Body Positive.* Retrieved May 11, 2009 from http://www.thebody.com/content/art30995.html

Smith, R. A. & Siplon, P. D. (2006). *Drugs into bodies: Global AIDS treatment activism.* Westport, Conn: Praeger.

Sontag, S. (1989). *AIDS and its metaphors.* London: Anchor Books.

Sontag, S. (1989). *Illness as metaphor.* New York: Picador USA.

Staff. (1997, December). The twilight of eradication: Infectious HIV persists after up to 2 1/2 years of triple drug therapy. *TAGline.* Retrieved March 17, 2009, from http://www.thebody.com/content/art1418.html#eradicate

Staff. (1997, July). Critically needed information on HIV/AIDS treatment adherence" *PI Perspective.* Retrieved March 20, 2009, from http://www.projectinform.org/press/1997/071097.shtml

Staff. (1999, Summer). Against the odds one man's battle against HIV, depression, & OI's. *Seattle Treatment Education Project.* Retrieved March 26, 2009, from http://www.thebody.com/content/treat/art1852.html

Staff. (2000, April). Alternatives 2000. *POZ Magazine*, (58). Retrieved March 29, 2009, from http://www.poz.com/articles/200_10451.shtml

Staff. (2001, June). It's a small AIDS world after all. *POZ Magazine,* 71. Retrieved May 14, 2009 from http://www.poz.com/articles/189_1183.shtml

Staff. (2004, May). The POZ decade-1996. *POZ Magazine.* Retrieved March 13, 2009, from http://www.poz.com/articles/154_277.shtml

Staff. (2004, May). The POZ decade-1997. *POZ Magazine.* Retrieved March 13, 2009, from http://www.poz.com/articles/154_279.shtml

Staff. (2004, May). The POZ decade-1998. *POZ Magazine.* Retrieved March 13, 2009, from http://www.poz.com/articles/154_280.shtml

Staff. (2007, March 14). Abbott to Thailand: No more drugs for you. *POZ Magazine News.* Retrieved May 20, 2009 from http://www.poz.com/articles/1_11516.shtml

Strub, S. (1996, August/September). S.O.S. *POZ Magazine,* (16). Retrieved March 29, 2009, from http://www.poz.com/articles/253_5194.shtml

Strub, S. (1997, April). S.O.S. *POZ Magazine,* (22), 12.

Strub, S. (1997, March). S.O.S. *POZ Magazine,* (152). Retrieved June 11, 2009, from http://www.poz.com/articles/238_12486.shtml

Strub, S. (2005, December 5). What's wrong with our movement. *POZ Magazine,* Retrieved June 11, 2009, from http://www.poz.com/articles/401_2411.shtml

Strub, S. (2008, September). Renewing the Denver Principles. *POZ Magazine,* Retrieved December, 12 2009 from http://www.poz.com/articles/sean_strub_usca_hiv_401_15335.shtml

Sullivan, A. (1996, November 10). When plagues end. *New York Times Magazine.* Retrieved March 2, 2009, from http://query.nytimes.com/gst/fullpage.html?res=9900E4DD1F39F933A25752C1A960958260

Summers, D. (1987) Sex in the eighties. In M. Callen's (Ed) *Surviving and thriving with AIDS: Hints for the newly diagnosed* (pp. 67-79). New York: People with AIDS Coalition.

Szymanski, K. (2000, October). The boys in the band. *POZ Magazine,* 64. Retrieved May 28, 2009 from http://www.poz.com/articles/206_1387.shtml

Terson, A. (1989, November). All about Alice. *Body Positive,* 2(8), 9.

Timour, K. (1997, May). Protease inhibitors — work, money, food, sex, and doctors: Seven myths examined. *Body Positive.* Retrieved May 7, 2009 from http://thebody.com/content/art30655.html

Timour, K. (1999, September). The Eleventh International Conference on AIDS — An activist perspective. *Body Positive*, p. 18.

Tips from long term survivors. (1989, September). *Vancouver People with AIDS Coalition Newsletter*, (24), 1.

Travers, R., Wilson, M. G., Flicker, S., Guta, A., Bereket, T., McKay, C., Rourke, S. B.(2008). The greater involvement of people living with AIDS principle: theory versus practice in Ontario's HIV/AIDS community-based research sector. *AIDS Care,* 20(6), 615-624.

Treatment Action Campaign. (2000). *Global march for HIV/AIDS treatment.* Retrieved May 19, 2009 from http://www.actupny.org/reports/durban-march.html

Treatment Action Group (n.d.) *Treatment Action Group.* Retrieved December 1, 2009 from http://www.thebody.com/content/art1512.html

Treatment Action Group. (2000, September). Being there. *Tagline.* Retrieved May 7, 2009 from ERLINK" http://www.thebody.com/content/world/art1546.html"

Treatment Action Group. (2000, September). Taking it to the street. *Tagline.* Retrieved November 28, 2009 from http://www.thebody.com/content/world/art1547.html

Treatment Action Group. (2004, September). The irony of Bangkok. *Tagline.* Retrieved May 28, 2009 from http://www.thebody.com/content/art1526.html

Treatment Action Group. (2008, Summer). Meet the activists: Battling the TB/HIV epidemic through community action. *TAGline.* Retrieved May 14, 2009 from http://www.thebody.com/content/art49275.html

Treichler, P. (1987). AIDS, homophobia, and biomedical discourse: An epidemic of signification. In D. Crimp (Ed.), *AIDS: Cultural analysis, cultural activism* (31-70). Boston: MIT Press.

Tuller, D. (2003, January). Generation next. *POZ Magazine,* 88. Retrieved May 14, 2009 from http://www.poz.com/articles/174_753.shtml

UNAIDS. (2008). Greater involvement of people living with or affected by HIV/AIDS (GIPA). UNAIDS. Retrieved December 10, 2009 from http://www.unaids.org/en/PolicyAndPractice/GIPA/default.asp

U.S. Centers for Disease Control and Prevention. (2001, April). HIV/AIDS drug ads blamed for unsafe sex. *CDC HIV/Hepatitis/STD/TB Prevention News Update.* Retrieved March 4, 2009, from http://www.thebody.com/content/art22990.html

Villarosa, L., Ickes, B., Scott, L., Joseph, N., Terrell, K., & Wortman, J. (2006, December). 35 ones to watch. *POZ Magazine,* 130. Retrieved May 28, 2009 from http://www.poz.com/articles/1891_10868.shtml

Watney, S. (1987). *Policing desire: AIDS, pornography, and the media*. London: Methuen.

Wilkinson, S. & Kitzinger, C. (1993). Whose breast is it anyway? A feminist consideration of advice and "treatment" for breast cancer. *Women's Studies Forum, 16*(3), 229-238.

Wilson, P. (1999, July). Inside Africa: Guest editor's letter. *POZ Magazine,* 49. Retrieved May 13, 2009, from http://www.poz.com/articles/216_10371.shtml

Withorn, A. (1980). Helping ourselves: The limits and potential of self-help. *Social-Policy,* 11(3), 20-27.

Women Alive. (2009). *Index of articles from Women Alive*. Retrieved May 25, 2009, from http://www.thebody.com/content/art56.html

Wong, W. T. & Ussher, J. M. (2008). Life with HIV and AIDS in the era of effective treatments: "It's not just about living longer!" *Social Theory & Health.* 6(2), 117-131.

World AIDS Campaign. (2008). World AIDS Day — Monday, 1 December 2008 media fact sheet. *World AIDS Campaign.* Retrieved May 4, 2009, from http://www.thebody.com/content/art49462.html

Wortman, J. (2009, April). Cut, print, it's a wrap! *POZ Magazine,* (153). Retrieved June 11, 2009, from http://www.poz.com/articles/ sex_positive_hiv_2311_16285.shtml

Wright, K., Cairns, G., Kaplan, E., Lederer, B., & Scondras, D. (2000, October). Conference of the century. *POZ Magazine,* 64. Retrieved May 7, 2009 from http://www.poz.com/articles/206_7784.shtml

Wychules, P. (1989, July/August). From the executive director. *Body Positive,* 2(6), 4.

Your brighter future starts here. (2009, May). *POZ Magazine,* (154). Retrieved October 30, 2009, from http://www.poz.com/articles/denver_principles_ future_hiv_2326_16506.shtml

ACKNOWLEDGMENTS

In writing this book I have relied on the support, patience and guidance of a great number of people — too many to mention in a simple, short acknowledgment. I am greatly indebted to them all and apologize if having overlooked expressing my gratitude. With regard to the origin of this project, I owe a great debt to Charles Roy for introducing me to organizing and activism among people with HIV/AIDS and the PWA movement. Without his foresight and guidance this book would not have been imaginable. Moreover, this book would not have been possible without the contributions of people with HIV/AIDS who have written about their lives and the epidemic in PWA media. The staff and volunteers at numerous AIDS organizations and PWA coalitions have been indispensable, especially Body Positive (New York), the AIDS Committee of Toronto, the British Columbia Persons with AIDS Society, the Hamilton AIDS Network, Community AIDS Treatment Information Exchange, members of the collective, The Positive Side, the writers and editors involved in Diseased Pariah News, and the people at POZ Magazine.

Among my colleagues, I wish to thank members of the McMaster HIV/AIDS Social Research Group: Roy Cain, Dorothy Pawluch, Dale Guenter and Rob Travers. Also, I am indebted to Barry Adam at the Department of Sociology and Anthropology at the University of Windsor for his insight and guidance. All the projects I manage to complete have been shaped and influenced by the mentorship of Peter Donnelly and Graham Knight, and this one is no exception. I also want to thank Phil, Brian, Mike, Sammi, Nancy, Chris, Art and Eric for their ongoing friendship and encouragement. Sections of this book were written while on research leave at the University of Otago in Wellington, New Zealand. The staff and colleagues along with the friends we met in Wellington and Dunedin were gracious hosts. I want to specifically thank Kevin Dew and Steve Jackson for their insightful commentary on the book. Over the years many research assistants and friends have helped with research and editing; I want to especially thank Nadia, Steph, Vass and Laura. To Justine, thanks for your careful editing and thoughtful feedback. I would like to acknowledge the support of the Social Sciences and Humanities Research Council and the Ontario HIV Treatment Exchange. And thanks to Dave Demers for supporting this project and preparing the manuscript for publication.

Most of all, I want to acknowledge the contribution of my family — Meghan, Hannah and Rebecca — for their love and care, and for giving me the inspiration and the time to complete this manuscript during our travels and adventures together. And last, I want to thank my parents, Robert and Margaret, for teaching me to believe that anything is possible.

INDEX

ABOUT THE AUTHOR

JAMES GILLETT is an associate professor at McMaster University in Hamilton, Ontario, Canada. He is jointly appointed in the Sociology Department and the Department of Health, Aging and Society. Dr. Gillett is a member of the McMaster HIV/AIDS Social Research Group. He has been a volunteer at the Hamilton AIDS Network, the AIDS Committee of Toronto and the Community AIDS Treatment Information Exchange.